A P
Work
Resi

A Primer on Working with Resistance

Martha Stark, M.D.

JASON ARONSON INC.
Northvale, New Jersey
London

Production Editor: Judith D. Cohen

This book was set in 11 pt. Times by Lind Graphics of Upper Saddle River, New Jersey, and printed and bound by Haddon Craftsmen of Scranton, Pennsylvania.

Copyright © 1994 by Jason Aronson Inc.

10   9   8   7   6   5   4   3   2   1

All rights reserved. Printed in the United States of America. No part of this book may be used or reproduced in any manner whatsoever without written permission from Jason Aronson Inc. except in the case of brief quotations in reviews for inclusion in a magazine, newspaper, or broadcast.

Library of Congress Cataloging-in-Publication Data

Stark, Martha.
    A primer on working with resistance / Martha Stark.
      p.   cm.
    Includes bibliographical references and index.
    ISBN 1-56821-093-0
    1. Resistance (Psychoanalysis)   2. Psychotherapist and patient.
    3. Transference (Psychology)   I. Title.
      [DNLM: 1. Conflict (Psychology)   2. Transference (Psychology)
    3. Psychoanalytic Therapy—methods.   BF 683 S795p   1994]
RC489.R49S729   1994
616.89'17—dc20
DNLM/DLC
for Library of Congress   93-32471

Manufactured in the United States of America. Jason Aronson Inc. offers books and cassettes. For information and catalog write to Jason Aronson Inc., 230 Livingston Street, Northvale, New Jersey 07647.

To Gunnar

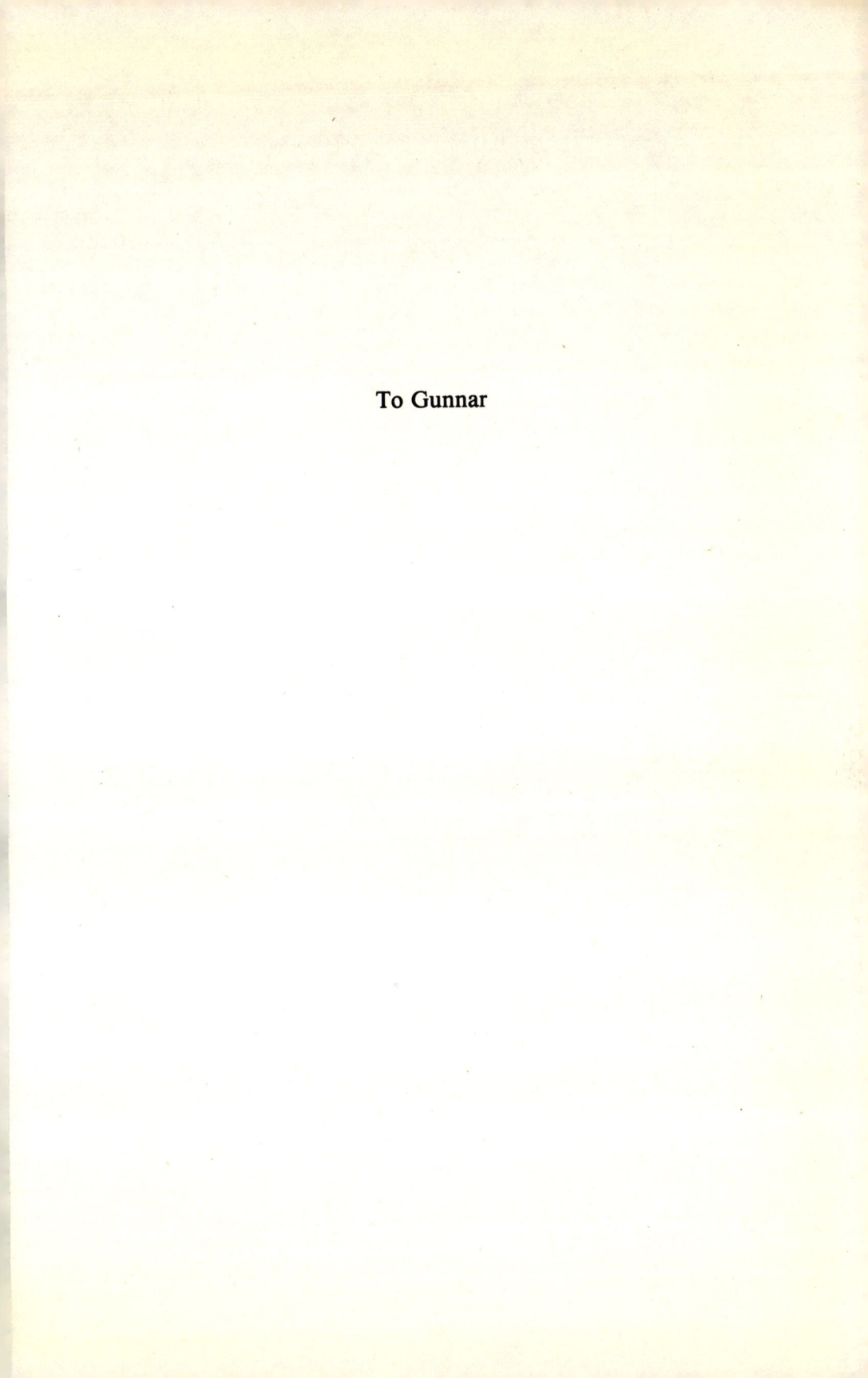

Contents

Foreword by David E. Scharff, M.D.   xxi

Preface   xxv

PART I
UNDERSTANDING RESISTANCE

1 The Concept of Resistance   3

    How does conflict manifest itself clinically?   3
    How does classical psychoanalysis conceptualize conflict?   4
    What are some examples of such conflicts?   4
    Why and how does the ego defend itself?   5
    How might we operationalize the concept of conflict?   5
    What are some more examples of conflict?   5
    In the final analysis, conflict involves tension between what kinds of forces?   6
    Are we addressing convergent or divergent conflict?   7

How is convergent conflict experienced by the patient?   8
How do knowledge and experience of reality relate to accuracy of perception?   8
What is meant by illusion and distortion?   8
How do illusion and distortion relate to the transference?   9
What is the nature of the patient's investment in his illusions and his distortions?   9
How do we reconcile the patient's fear of the bad object with his need for it?   10
What is the relationship between the patient's transference and his capacity to experience reality?   10
What constitutes mental health?   11
What are the numbers of ways we can describe conflict?   12
What creates anxiety?   12
What eases anxiety?   13
Is the distinction between intrapsychic and interpersonal clinically useful?   13
How does conflict relate to reality and defense?   14
What is the relationship between defense and resistance?   14
What is the difference between toxic and nontoxic reality?   15
What, then, is the resistance?   17

2 Resistance as Failure to Grieve   19

What does the child do when faced with the unbearably painful reality of the parental limitations?   19
How does internalizing the parental badness apply to survivors of abuse?   20
How do early-on toxic failures create the need for illusion and distortion?   20
What is the relationship, then, between the failure to grieve and the need for defense?   21
What do we mean by the repetition compulsion?   22
How does it come to pass that the repetition compulsion has such a profound impact on what we feel and do?   22
How does the repetition compulsion relate to the wish for containment?   23
How does the repetition compulsion both hinder and help?   23
How does the treatment situation create the opportunity to grieve?   24
What is the relationship between grieving and the repetition compulsion?   24
What does it mean to grieve?   24
What is pseudo-grief?   25

CONTENTS

How does the patient's experience of internal impoverishment speak to his failure to grieve? 26
What is the refrain of the patient with unmourned losses? 26
What is involved in therapeutic impasses? 27
More generally, how does the patient's failure to grieve relate to the resistance? 28

3 Mastering Resistance by Way of Grieving 29

What must the patient come to understand before he can move on? 29
What is the role of grieving with respect to the early-on parental failures? 30
What is the relationship between grieving and internalizing? 30
How does working through the transference involve relinquishing the defenses? 31
How is paradox involved? 31
How does working through the transference involve grieving? 31
How does resolving the transference promote the patient's mental health? 32

4 Grieving, Internalization, and Development of Capacity 33

What is self psychology? 33
How does self psychology conceive of the relationship between grieving, internalization, and structuralization? 34
How does the patient become autonomous? 35
What is the distinction between nontraumatic (or optimal) and traumatic disillusionment? 35
Why is the distinction between nontraumatic and traumatic so crucial? 36
How does self psychology inform our understanding of the development of healthy structure? 36
What is meant by psychic structure (or capacity)? 37
How does self psychology inform our understanding of the process by which internal drive regulation develops? 38
How do we describe such a transformative process? 38
How are anal strivings transformed into healthy capacity? 38
How are oedipal strivings transformed into healthy capacity? 40
More generally, what is the result of taming id needs? 40
How does self psychology inform our understanding of the process by which internal self regulation develops? 41
What is the relationship between such transformations and working through the transference? 41

What happens to the need for a perfect self? 42
What happens to the need for a perfect object? 42
Are the internalized standards realistic or perfectionistic? 43
What are empty depressions? 44
What results from working through disrupted positive transferences? 44
What is the relationship between the patient's need for perfection and, more generally, his need for illusion? 45
What does it mean to develop mature capacity? 45
Why do we turn to self theory to inform our understanding of this transformative process? 46

5 Development of Pathology 47

What is the villain in this piece? 47
In order to understand the development of pathology, where should we start? 48
What do we mean by infantile need? 48
What are examples of such needs? 48
What happens when the child's infantile needs are traumatically frustrated? 49
With traumatic frustration, what happens to the infantile need? 49
What happens to traumatically thwarted anal needs? 49
What happens to traumatically thwarted oedipal needs? 50
What happens to traumatically thwarted narcissistic needs? 50
What are neurotic and narcissistic needs? 51
With traumatic frustration, what does not get internalized that should? 51
How are need and deficit related? 52
With traumatic frustration, what does get internalized that should not? 53
What does Fairbairn say about internalization and structuralization? 53
In summary, what are the three things that happen when there is traumatic frustration of an infantile need? 54
What, then, are we saying happens when there is the experience of bad against a backdrop of good? 55
What is the relationship between internalization and separation from the infantile object? 55
What exactly is the nature of the attachment to the internal bad object? 56
What is the clinical relevance of the patient's intense attachments to his internal bad objects? 56
How does Fairbairn help us understand such attachments? 57

CONTENTS

How do intense attachments to internal bad objects fuel the
    patient's resistance to relinquishing the infantile object?   59
What are pathogenic introjects?   59
What do we know about the patient's attachments to, and
    identifications with, his internal bad objects?   60
With respect to our understanding of internal bad objects,
    what does Freud have to say?   61
With respect to our understanding of internal bad objects,
    what does Fairbairn have to say?   62
What is Freud's contribution to our understanding of the
    relationship between internal bad objects?   63
What is Fairbairn's contribution to our understanding of the
    relationship between internal bad objects?   65
What do Kernberg and Meissner have to say about the
    relationship between internal bad objects?   65
What about the victimizer and victim introjective pair?   66
What about the superior and inferior introjective pair?   67
How do these introjective configurations relate
    to depression?   67
How does a two-person psychology conceive of conflict?   68
Is relational conflict thought to be convergent or divergent?   69
Traumatic frustration results in what kind of conflict?   69
Why does the patient have negative misperceptions of
    himself and others?   70

6 Working with the Transference   73

How does a negative transference develop?   73
What is a direct transference?   74
What is an inverted transference?   74
What is an example of an inverted transference?   75
How are negative transferences resolved?   75
How does a one-person theory conceive of resolution of the
    negative transference?   75
How does a two-person theory conceive of resolution of the
    negative transference?   76
What are the two internal records of traumatic frustrations?   77
How does this relate to the unfolding of the transference?   77
What is the relationship between positive and negative
    transference?   78
What is the relationship between positive transference
    and hope?   78
What is the relationship between negative transference
    and fear?   79
Which transferences do we interpret?   79

What is the distinction between a positive transference disrupted
   and a negative transference?   80
Why is such a distinction important?   81
What is an idealizing transference?   81
How are we to understand the processes by which new good is
   added and old bad is changed?   83
How does self psychology inform our understanding of structural
   growth?   83
How does object relations theory inform our understanding
   of structural change?   83
What are serial dilutions?   84
When, and to what extent, is the therapist (in his capacity
   as a transference object) experienced as a new good object or as
   an old bad one?   85
What is the deficiency-compensation model of therapeutic
   action?   85
What is the relational-conflict model of therapeutic action?   86
Why does the patient need both a new good object and an
   old bad one?   87

PART II
CLINICAL INTERVENTIONS

7 Listening to the Patient   91

Does the patient want to be understood or to understand?   91
Can you say more about when the patient wants
   to be understood?   92
What did Balint and Winnicott have to say about the
   therapist's stance in relation to the patient?   92
Can you say more about when the patient wants
   to understand?   93
How does the therapist decide whether the patient wants
   to be understood or to understand?   93
How does the therapist position himself in relation
   to the patient?   94
How does the therapist's stance in relation to the patient affect
   the level of the patient's anxiety?   94
How does the therapist engage the patient's experiencing ego
   and his observing ego?   94
What does working through the resistance mean?   95

CONTENTS

Does the therapist address himself to the present, the transference, or the past? 95
Why is it important that the therapist be able to decenter? 96
What is the distinction between easy empathy and difficult empathy? 96
What does it mean to be truly empathic? 97
How much are we with the patient where he is and how much do we direct his attention elsewhere? 98
What is the technical task for the therapist? 98
What about the recurring patterns and themes? 99
How do we highlight the patient as agent? 99

8 Responding to the Patient — 101

What are some fairly typical situations of conflict? 101
How do we challenge the patient's defense? 102
How do we support the patient's defense? 102
What happens if we first challenge and then support the patient's defense? 103
What, more specifically, does a conflict statement do? 104
What are examples of statements that simply support or reinforce the patient's resistance? 105
How does naming the patient's defense relate to defining the patient's characteristic stance in the world? 106
How do we attempt to empower the patient? 107
What is an example of supporting the patient's defense? 108
How can the therapist both convey his respect for the patient's need and highlight its defensive aspect? 109
How, then, does the therapist convey to the patient that he has been heard? 109
What is another example of supporting the patient's defense? 110
How does the conflict statement attempt to keep the conflict within the patient instead of between patient and therapist? 112
What does a defense-against-affect conflict statement address? 114
What are examples of defense-against-affect conflict statements? 115
What does the first part of the defense-against-affect conflict statement do? 117
What does the second part of the defense-against-affect conflict statement do? 117
Why is it important that the therapist address the level of the patient's knowledge of his conflict? 118

What is the difference between highlighting what the
   patient is feeling and highlighting what the patient knows
   he is feeling?   119
What is the difference between highlighting what the patient
   is feeling and highlighting what the patient knows he
   must be feeling?   119
What is the difference between highlighting what the patient
   is feeling and highlighting what the patient finds
   himself feeling?   120
Finally, what is the difference between highlighting what the
   patient is feeling and highlighting what the patient tells himself
   he feels?   120
In other words, how does the therapist make his interventions
   experience-near?   121
How does the defense-against-affect conflict statement both
   validate experience and enhance knowledge?   121
How do conflict statements, more generally, attempt to empower,
   validate experience, and enhance knowledge?   122
What is the structure of the conflict statement?   122
What stance does the therapist take in relation to the
   patient's conflict?   123
How do we convey our understanding of a patient's investment
   in an abusive relationship?   124
How do we hope the patient will respond to a conflict
   statement?   125
What are the realities against which the patient feels the
   need to defend himself?   126
What are the three different kinds of conflict statements
   corresponding to these realities?   126
More specifically, what does a price-paid conflict statement
   address?   127
What must the patient understand before he can relinquish
   the defense?   128
What does a work-to-be-done conflict statement address?   129
What, more generally, do conflict statements highlight?   130
In the following conflict statements, what does the patient
   defend against and what is doing the defending?   130
How does a conflict statement both confront the patient
   and paradox him?   132
What are examples of conflict statements that confront?   132
What are examples of conflict statements that paradox?   133
How does the therapist titrate the patient's anxiety?   134

CONTENTS

What is the optimal level of anxiety? 134
What is an inverted conflict statement? 135
To what extent does the therapist confront the defense, support the defense, or do both? 136
What is your own stylistic preference? 137
For conflict statements to be effective, what capacities must the patient have? 138
What is the classic example of a patient who lacks the capacity to tolerate internal conflict? 139
Instead of help with working through conflict, what does the borderline most need from the therapist? 140
What is a containing statement? 140
How does a containing statement bring the patient up short? 141
How, then, do conflict statements facilitate the patient's progress in the treatment? 142
What is a path-of-least-resistance statement? 143
What creates therapeutic impasses? 145
What is an example of a therapeutic impasse? 146
What kinds of interventions do we make when there is a therapeutic impasse? 146
What is a damaged-for-life statement? 147
What is a compensation statement? 148
What is an entitlement statement? 149
More generally, what happens when the patient's distortions, illusions, and entitlement get delivered into the relationship with the therapist? 150
What is an illusion statement? 152
How are illusion statements used to suggest disillusionment? 153
What is a disillusionment statement? 154
Is a disillusionment statement a particular kind of conflict statement? 155
What is an integration statement? 155
What is a distortion statement? 157
What is a legitimization statement? 159
What is a modification statement? 161
Is a modification statement a particular kind of conflict statement? 163
What is an inverted modification statement? 164
What is a facilitation statement? 165
Is a facilitation statement a particular kind of conflict statement? 167

PART III
CLINICAL PRACTICE

9 The Cocoon Transference 171

Is the transference an aspect of the resistance? 171
With what kind of power does the patient vest the therapist? 172
Why do patients resist delivering themselves and their vulnerabilities into the treatment situation? 173
What is the defense of affective nonrelatedness? 173
How is the patient conflicted in the initial stages of the treatment? 174
How does the therapist respond to the patient's denial of object need? 174
How does the therapist convey his appreciation for how invested the patient may be in his defenses? 175
How are facilitation statements useful? 176
How are legitimization statements useful? 176
How are work-to-be-done conflict statements useful? 177
How is the patient's affective nonengagement finally worked through? 178

10 The Positive Transference and Its Disruptions 179

How does the positive transference emerge? 179
What happens to frustrated need? 180
What is benevolent containment? 181
What is an important difference between psychological and physiological needs? 181
What are id needs and what are ego needs? 182
Why do we turn to self psychology? 182
How does a narcissistic patient with structural deficit initially present? 183
How does the patient's need for perfection manifest itself in the transference? 184
What do we mean by a second chance? 185
What is the role of illusion in a narcissistic transference? 185
What if the therapist's failures are traumatic ones? 186
How is the illusion statement useful? 186
What is the role of entitlement in a narcissistic transference? 187
How is the entitlement statement useful? 188
What is the defense of relentless entitlement? 189

How is the legitimization statement useful? 189
How do illusion, entitlement, and legitimization statements lay the groundwork for the eventual working through of the patient's disillusionment? 190
How does the patient respond to interventions that direct his attention away from where he is in the moment? 191
What happens when the therapist sermonizes? 191
What does it mean to comply with the patient's narcissistic demands? 192
How is gratification of need necessary but not sufficient for growth? 193
Why do we not interpret a positive transference? 193
Why do we interpret disrupted positive transferences? 194
What is the relationship between recognition of separateness and capacity to internalize? 194
What is a disrupted positive transference? 196
What is narcissistic rage? 197
How does the therapist locate the offending failure? 198
What is required of the therapist? 198
Is misperception involved in the patient's upset with the therapist? 199
Is not the positive transference a situation of seduction and betrayal? 200
How is the disillusionment statement useful? 202
How is the integration statement useful? 203
What must the patient grieve? 203
How is paradox involved? 204
What is involved in grieving his disenchantment? 205
How do self psychologists conceive of mental health? 206

11 The Negative Transference   207

Why do we turn from self psychology to object relations theory in order to understand the negative transference and its resolution? 207
Why is the distinction between the absence of good and the presence of bad so important? 208
What is the relationship between structural growth and structural change? 209
What are clinical examples of structural growth? 209
What are clinical examples of structural change? 210
What accompanies these transformations? 211
What are the therapeutic agents of change? 211

How does the therapist intervene when insight is the goal?
How does he intervene when a corrective experience
is the goal?   212
How is insight a corrective for transference distortion?   213
How is the relationship itself a corrective for
transference distortion?   214
How is paradox involved?   215
How does object relations theory inform our understanding
of how the negative transference is resolved?   216
How do we recognize the existence of a negative
transference?   218
What is the relationship between projection and transference
on the one hand and projective identification and
countertransference on the other?   218
How do direct transference, projection, and projective
identification relate to one another?   219
Is projective identification an instance of transference?   220
How do inverted transference, projection, and projective
identification relate to one another?   220
In this chapter on negative transference, what will our
focus be?   221
In a negative transference, where is the locus of control
and power?   222
What are the negative filters through which the patient
experiences himself and others?   222
How is the distortion statement useful?   223
How is the legitimization statement useful?   224
How does the therapist direct the patient's attention inward
and backward?   225
How does the achievement of insight foster change?   225
How does the therapist direct the patient's attention
outward?   226
How can the modification statement be useful?   227
How can the inverted modification statement be useful?   228
What happens as the patient begins to experience the
therapist as a new good object?   230
What is the role of grieving in resolving the negative
transference?   230
How does the defense become increasingly ego-dystonic?   231
What is the role of the synthetic function of the ego?   231
How does separation from the infantile object relate to
overcoming the resistance?   232

CONTENTS

    What is the relationship between empathy and projective identification?   232
    Why is it so difficult for the therapist to get it just right?   234

12 The Attainment of Mature Hope   235

    How is unrealistic hope transformed into realistic hope?   235

References   237

Index   241

Foreword

Martha Stark's primer on resistance is a unique book. It takes as the heart of the clinical problem the patient's reluctance to change—that ubiquitous and paradoxical phenomenon of our work in which people come to us asking for help in changing, and then do their level best to keep change from happening. Freud noticed this problem from the beginning, and located the necessity to confront resistance as the central problem of technique. Soon he joined that discovery with that of the transference, making the work with transference and resistance the hallmark of psychoanalytic technique.

Much of classical psychoanalytic and psychotherapeutic training in North America has followed Freud in placing work with resistance at the center of technique. The dictum "First interpret the resistance, and only then the impulse," has characterized the mainstream of training in this country for many years, in contrast to the technical suppositions of the British schools of Klein and object relations, which emphasized the use of the transference, often encouraging early interpretation of the transference equally on the side of the resistance born out of fear and the wish born out of neediness. The Kleinians particularly emphasized the importance of understanding the patient's aggressive and libidinal approach to the therapist from the beginning of the process, teaching that early interpretation of these elements could bypass the patient's resistant fear and offer superior results therapeutically.

On this side of the Atlantic, Kohut's self psychology offered another challenge to the classical American line of thought and practice. His emphasis on the need for therapist empathy for the patient seemed to shift emphasis away from the analysis of resistance, and toward the repair of deficit in the patient's experience, toward the patient's need for the therapist to be a compliant "selfobject," serving the patient rather than confronting, subserving need rather than understanding conflict.

These two developments combine to make a reexamination of the central concepts and tenets of ego psychology a crucial undertaking. Ego psychology is still the central orientation in American psychoanalysis and analytic psychotherapy, although the influence from these other schools is increasingly manifest. We can no longer accept the old tenets of theory or practice without question, for they are being questioned by both friendly and unfriendly critics. Does this mean they have little or no meaning? Or can we undertake the task of reexamination and refinement to improve and clarify the essential contribution that the old conveyed?

It is obvious from my question that I believe we should and can do this work, but as important as it is, it is difficult. It requires that those who would undertake such a task steep themselves in the new contributions without abandoning the old, look for the similarities and differences with a critical but open mind, and do the painful work of synthesizing from a position of flexibility and openness rather than take the easier path of making choices on the basis of early loyalty and unexamined personal preference.

Martha Stark has contributed a powerful beginning to this process. In her longer volume on resistance, she has examined the theoretical underpinnings of these processes, but in this volume she has done something even more unusual: she has defined specifically the refinements to technique that follow from her theoretical examination. "Here," she says, "one can usefully say this, and there, we can suggest another approach." This specificity is not only useful to

FOREWORD

the novice therapist. It enables the experienced practitioner and teacher to follow her argument down to its practical consequence, to see clearly the implication of her argument, and to agree or disagree with an equal specificity—that is, to engage in a thoughtful counterpoint.

Along the way to this achievement, Dr. Stark has examined and synthesized a great deal. While her background and training are centered in ego psychology, she has studied and absorbed the teachings of Kohut and Klein, of Winnicott and Fairbairn. She brings the lessons of these theorists and contributors to bear as she enlarges the notion of working with resistance to formulate a compleat approach to psychotherapy, one consistent with classical psychoanalytic psychotherapy, but enriched and enlarged by the wisdom she has acquired in her broader travels. What emerges is a work that is a specific guide, but one that does not suffer from oversimplification or narrow-mindedness. This is a work which is at once a practical guide and a theoretical tour de force. Readers who journey in this slim volume with Dr. Stark will return from their travels to their practice much educated, having encountered new ideas and old ones in new forms, better able to face the everyday travails of psychotherapy.

—David E. Scharff, M.D.

Preface

I once attended a seminar at which the speaker, in response to a query from the audience, quipped: "Now *that's* a good question. A good question is a question to which I know the answer!" This may well be what a good question is, and certainly we all like to be asked such questions.

But a *really* good question is one that challenges, stimulates, and provokes—a question that you may not initially be able to answer or that may require considerable thought in order to be answered with integrity.

Jason Aronson was the inspiration for *A Primer on Working with Resistance,* a book that contains many questions, some of which are good ones and some of which are really good ones. After Dr. Aronson read the final manuscript of my first book, *Working with Resistance,* he said he thought the material presented in that book would lend itself nicely to a question-and-answer format; such a format would provide the serious reader with a clear, crisp, concise, and compact guide to working with resistant patients.

He offered me the opportunity to write a second book, a companion guide to the first, that would systematically organize the theoretical constructs as well as their clinical applications in such a way as to make them accessible to a broad range of mental health practitioners, from the beginning student to the more advanced clinician.

Writing this primer has been a wonderfully exhilarating but extremely challenging project; it is not easy to take fairly complex theoretical and clinical issues and refine them, tease out their essence, pare them down to their most basic and purest form—so that the ideas can be readily grasped by the practitioner and usefully applied to the clinical situation.

I begin with the claim that the resistant patient is a patient who has not been able to confront the reality of past and present losses, disappointments, and frustrations, who instead protects himself from the pain of his grief by clinging to his defenses. The resistant patient is a defended patient within whom there is conflict, conflict between those healthy forces that press "Yes" and those unhealthy (resistive) counterforces that insist "No." The resistant patient is a defended patient is a conflicted patient, who resists feeling what (he knows) he should feel and resists doing what (he knows) he should do.

I go on to integrate concepts drawn from classical psychoanalysis, self psychology, and object relations theory, in order to present a contemporary theory of therapeutic action that takes into consideration structural conflict, structural deficit, and relational conflict—all of which, ultimately, fuel the patient's resistance, impede the patient's progress in the treatment, and oppose the patient's movement toward health and the realization of his potential. The emphasis is always upon how theory informs clinical practice.

My first book, *Working with Resistance,* develops many of the ideas presented here in greater depth and elaborates, in particular, upon the defense of relentless entitlement, a defense against grieving to which patients with underlying sadomasochistic dynamics cling with incredible tenacity. In my first book, in order to demonstrate the actual working through of various resistances, I also present some process recordings and discuss, at length, five specific clinical situations.

PREFACE

I would like to thank Dr. Aronson for his very generous and enthusiastic support; his wise encouragement to "ride the horse in the direction it's going" has allowed me to deliver my most authentic and most creative self into my writing. I would also like to express my heartfelt gratitude to Dr. Sheldon Roth, who has been a constant source of inspiration; his faith in me has meant the world to me.

I am extremely grateful to all my students and supervisees, who, over the course of the past years, have had the ability and the courage to ask me those really good questions and have had the capacity to tolerate my not always knowing, right away, the answers.

Writing this primer was a deeply satisfying experience that demanded the best of me; my hope is that the reader will enjoy it, will himself be challenged by it, and will find it to be a convenient and accessible resource guide to working with resistance.

Author's note: In the interest of simplicity and uniformity, I have decided to avoid the awkward and confusing reference to "he/she" and "him/her." In this book, therefore, everyone is referred to as "he."

I

Understanding Resistance

1

Understanding Resistance

ONE

The Concept of Resistance

How Does Conflict Manifest Itself Clinically?

Every day after work, a very depressed young man sits in the dark in his living room hour after hour, doing nothing, his mind blank. By his side is his stereo and a magnificent collection of his favorite classical music. The flick of a switch and he would feel better—and yet night after night, overwhelmed with despair, he just sits, never once touching that switch.

I would like to suggest that we think of this man as being in a state of internal conflict (although he may not, at this point, be aware of such conflict). He could turn on his stereo, but he does not. He could do something that would make him feel better, but he does nothing. Within this man is tension between what he "should" let himself do and what he finds himself doing instead.

In general, patients both do and don't want to get better. They both do and don't want to maintain things as they are. They both do and don't want to get on with their lives. They both are and aren't invested in their suffering. They are truly conflicted about all the choices that confront them.

The patient may protest that he desperately wants to change. He does and he doesn't. He may insist that he would do anything in order to feel better. Well, yes and no. On some level, everybody wants things to be better, but few are willing to change.

HOW DOES CLASSICAL PSYCHOANALYSIS CONCEPTUALIZE CONFLICT?

Drive theory conceives of conflict as involving internal tension between id impulse insisting "yes" and ego defense protesting "no" (with the superego coming down usually on the side of the ego). In Ralph Greenson's (1967) words: "A neurotic conflict is an unconscious conflict between an id impulse seeking discharge and an ego defense warding off the impulse's direct discharge or access to consciousness" (p. 17).

Although drives are considered part of the id, affects (drive derivatives) are thought to reside in the ego; in fact, the ego is said to be the seat of all affects. When Freud writes of psychic conflict between the id and the ego, it is understood that sometimes he is referring to conflict between an id drive and an ego defense and sometimes he is referring to conflict between an anxiety-provoking affect (in the ego but deriving from the id) and an ego defense.

WHAT ARE SOME EXAMPLES OF SUCH CONFLICTS?

The patient is sad but does not let himself cry.

The patient is angry but is determined to remain in control.

The patient is upset but tries not to let it show.

The patient is frightened but pretends he is not.

The patient is disappointed but claims that all is well.

WHY AND HOW DOES THE EGO DEFEND ITSELF?

In each of the above situations, the patient is experiencing some affect that makes him feel anxious or uncomfortable. But he does not like feeling that way and so defends himself against the feeling by denying its existence, by protesting that he does not feel that way, or by insisting that he feels something else altogether; in any of a number of ways, the patient defends himself against the anxiety-provoking or painful affect.

In each instance, the patient is experiencing an affect that the ego finds intolerable. In order to defend itself against the anxiety aroused by the affect, the ego mobilizes a defense to oppose the affect.

The net result is conflict, variously described as neurotic, intrapsychic, or structural.

HOW MIGHT WE OPERATIONALIZE THE CONCEPT OF CONFLICT?

Let us think, more generally, of psychic conflict as speaking to tension within the patient between those healthy forces that press "Yes" and those unhealthy counterforces that insist "No."

For example, there is always tension within the patient between his recognition that it is up to him to take responsibility for his life (which speaks to his healthy wish to get better) and his conviction that it should not have to be his responsibility (which speaks to his unhealthy need to preserve things as they are). There is always tension within the patient between his healthy investment in changing and his unhealthy reluctance to let go of his old ways of doing things.

WHAT ARE SOME MORE EXAMPLES OF CONFLICT?

The patient would like to do well on his examination, and yet he just can't seem to make himself study.

The patient knows that he should talk about how angry he is with his father, but he does not yet feel ready to do that.

The patient knows that he should try to come on time to his sessions, but he finds himself consistently arriving 5 to 10 minutes into the hour.

The patient wants to remember his dreams, but he is unwilling to write them down.

The patient knows that he has paid a steep price for having had such an emotionally abusive mother, but he is not yet prepared to deal with that.

On some level the patient knows that eventually he must deal with just how disappointed he is in his therapist, but he is hoping that he'll be able to get better without having to do that.

The patient wants to succeed, but he is not entirely sure that he deserves to make it.

The patient knows that his therapist doesn't really have all the answers, but he wishes his therapist did.

In his heart of hearts the patient knows that his mother will never really love him as he wants to be loved, and yet he finds himself continuing to hope that maybe someday she will.

The patient knows that he must be sad about the death of his father, but he can't seem to let himself really feel it.

IN THE FINAL ANALYSIS, CONFLICT INVOLVES TENSION BETWEEN WHAT KINDS OF FORCES?

Ultimately, the force defended against is the healthy (but anxiety-provoking) force within each of us that empowers us to change, the force that empowers us to relinquish our ties to the past in order to get on with the present, the force that empowers us to move forward in our lives. The counterforce is the unhealthy (but anxiety-assuaging) force within each of us that resists change, the force that clings tenaciously to the past, the force that impedes our progress in life.

In the final analysis, conflict involves tension between the patient's healthy wish to change and his unhealthy resistance to change.

ARE WE ADDRESSING CONVERGENT OR DIVERGENT CONFLICT?

Because we are here discussing the patient's resistance, our interest is in convergent conflict (Kris 1977), conflict between two opposing forces, one force originating as a defense against the other, in fact depending upon the other for its very existence. Convergent conflict arises in the context of tension between one force that presses "Yes" and another force that opposes with a "No." The conflict between force and counterforce is known as a conflict of defense or convergent conflict.

For example, consider an aggressive impulse that is opposed by the force of repression. The presence of the id aggression arouses anxiety in the ego, which prompts the ego to mobilize a defense. The repressive force is a direct result of the presence of the aggression. This is an instance, therefore, of convergent conflict.

When drive theorists speak of psychic conflict, they are usually referring to "intersystemic" conflict between id impulse (or derivative affect) and ego defense—that is, convergent conflict between forces within separate psychic structures (or systems).

By comparison, there are "intrasystemic" conflicts between forces within the same psychic structure, be it the id, the ego, or the superego. There is conflict, for example, between love and hate, active and passive, love of one's country and love of one's family, fear of failure and fear of success, to name a few. These are divergent conflicts.

Divergent conflict arises from conflict between two forces that are mutually exclusive. No longer are we talking about two forces in a state of dynamic equilibrium; now we are talking about two forces vying for exclusivity. Either the one or the other will triumph.

In what follows, we will be addressing ourselves primarily to the convergent conflict that exists between two forces in direct opposition to each other, the one a defense against the other. More specifically, we will be concerned with the patient's experience of the tension within him between the two forces in opposition. It will be this internal tension that will eventually provide the impetus for overcoming the patient's resistance.

HOW IS CONVERGENT CONFLICT EXPERIENCED BY THE PATIENT?

On the one hand, the patient has some awareness of what he "should" be feeling/doing; he has some knowledge of what is "right" or "healthy." On the other hand, he finds himself feeling/doing something other than that. On some level, the patient always knows the truth; on another level, he finds himself defending against the acknowledgment of it.

Expressed in somewhat different terms, there is ever tension within the patient between what he knows to be real and what he experiences as real—in other words, tension between his knowledge of reality and his experience of it.

HOW DO KNOWLEDGE AND EXPERIENCE OF REALITY RELATE TO ACCURACY OF PERCEPTION?

The patient's knowledge of reality has to do with accurate perception, with the ability to perceive things as they really are, uncontaminated by the need for them to be otherwise.

The patient's experience of reality, however, often has more to do with inaccurate perception deriving from early-on experiences with the parental object.

WHAT IS MEANT BY ILLUSION AND DISTORTION?

The patient's misperceptions of reality are either unrealistically positive, which I will refer to as *illusions,* or unrealistically negative, which I will refer to as *distortions.*

Even though on some level the patient knows better, he is nonetheless always misinterpreting the present, making assumptions about the present based on the past. Because of parental neglect and abuse early on, the patient now looks to his contemporary objects to be the good parent he never had (illusion) and/or expects them to be the bad parent he did have (distortion).

Whether illusion or distortion, the patient clings to his misperceptions of his objects in order not to have to know the truth about them. Whether such objects are past or present, the patient holds fast to defenses that protect him from having to confront his knowledge of who his objects really are.

HOW DO ILLUSION AND DISTORTION RELATE TO THE TRANSFERENCE?

The illusions and the distortions to which the patient clings in order not to have to know the truth about his objects fuel the transference — both the positive transference (in which the patient's "wish for good" is delivered into the treatment situation and the patient comes to hope that the therapist will be the good parent he never had) and the negative transference (in which the patient's "fear of bad" is delivered into the treatment situation and the patient comes to fear that the therapist will be the bad parent he did have).

WHAT IS THE NATURE OF THE PATIENT'S INVESTMENT IN HIS ILLUSIONS AND HIS DISTORTIONS?

Quite understandably, the patient very much needs the therapist to be the good parent he never had so that he can get now what he never got then.

But the patient also needs the therapist to be the bad parent he did have so that he does not have to face the intolerably painful reality that things could be, and could therefore have been, different.

In other words, even though the patient fears that the therapist will turn out to be bad (like the parent), he also needs the therapist to be bad so that he will not have to confront the reality that things need not have been as bad as they were. On some level, it is easier for the patient to experience the therapist as bad than to let in the anxiety-provoking truth that the therapist is not.

Acknowledging the reality that the therapist is not as bad as the patient had assumed he would be makes the patient intolerably anxious because it so threatens his attachment to the parent; similarly, confronting the reality that things could be, and could therefore have been, different poses a serious challenge to the patient's characteristic ways of experiencing his objects (and himself in relation to his objects).

And so it is that the patient both needs his therapist to be the good parent he never had (in order to compensate for the damage sustained early on) and needs his therapist to be the bad parent he did have (so that his loyalty to the parent will not be jeopardized).

HOW DO WE RECONCILE THE PATIENT'S FEAR OF THE BAD OBJECT WITH HIS NEED FOR IT?

Although consciously the patient fears the bad object, unconsciously he has a need for it. In other words, the patient's fear of bad is experience-near and his need for bad is experience-distant.

WHAT IS THE RELATIONSHIP BETWEEN THE PATIENT'S TRANSFERENCE AND HIS CAPACITY TO EXPERIENCE REALITY?

When a positive transference arises, tension is created within the patient between his knowledge of reality and his need for illusion. For example, the therapist does not have all the answers and, on some level, the patient knows this, but the patient nonetheless finds himself continuing to hope that the therapist does.

When a negative transference arises, tension is created within the patient between his knowledge of reality and his need for distortion. For example, the therapist will not laugh at the patient and, on some level, the patient knows this (because the therapist has never laughed at him), but the patient nonetheless finds himself fearing that the therapist might.

There is tension within the patient, therefore, between his healthy ability to experience the therapist as he is and his transferential need to experience the therapist as he is not. There is always tension within the patient between his recognition of the reality that his therapist is not the good parent he would have wanted him to be and his need to believe that he is (or will turn out to be). By the same token, there is always tension within the patient between his recognition of the reality that his therapist is not the bad parent he had imagined him to be and his need to believe that he is (or will turn out to be).

There is ever conflict within the patient between his recognition of reality and his need for illusion, between his recognition of reality and his need for distortion, and between reality (which the patient on some level does know, even though he sometimes chooses to forget) and illusion/distortion (to which the patient clings in order not to have to know the truth).

The tension is between the patient's healthy ability to experience his objects as they really are and his transferential need to experience them as they are not — in other words, the tension is between reality and transference.

To put it more generally, there is always tension within the patient between his capacity to experience reality as it is and his need to experience it as it is not.

WHAT CONSTITUTES MENTAL HEALTH?

There are, of course, numerous ways to define mental health. I would like to propose a definition that emphasizes the patient's capacity to experience reality as it is, uncontaminated by the need for it to be otherwise. Mental health has to do, then, with the capacity to experience one's objects as they really are, uncontaminated by the need for them to be other than who they are; it speaks to the ability to accept objects as they are, needing them to be neither better nor worse than they actually are.

Mental illness could thus be seen as the inability (or perhaps unwillingness) to experience one's objects as they really are. The patient who, early on, was traumatically disappointed at the hands of his parent will, as an adult, have both the intense wish for his objects to be the good parent he never had and the desperate fear that they will turn out to be the bad parent he did have (even as he is needing it to be that way). These wishes and fears contaminate subsequent relationships and make it difficult for the patient to perceive his objects as they really are; these wishes and fears, therefore, constitute his pathology.

It follows, then, that the greater the patient's capacity to experience reality as it is, the healthier he will be; the healthier the patient, the greater his capacity to know reality and to accept it. By the same token, the stronger the patient's need to experience reality as it is not, the more conflicted and the more resistant he will be; the more stuck the patient, the more powerful will be his need to experience his objects as different from who they really are.

WHAT ARE THE NUMBERS OF WAYS WE CAN DESCRIBE CONFLICT?

To this point, we have variously described conflict as the tension existing within the patient between drive (or drive derivative) and defense, id and ego, healthy force that presses "Yes" and unhealthy counterforce that insists "No," new and old, present and past, wish to change and resistance to change, knowledge and experience, capacity to know and need not to know, accurate perception and misperception, reality and transference, mental health and pathology. Although each pair speaks to a different way of conceptualizing conflict, what all pairs have in common is tension within them between something that creates anxiety and something that eases it.

Let us look, then, at both the thing that provokes anxiety and the thing that assuages it.

WHAT CREATES ANXIETY?

The thing that creates anxiety is an anxiety-provoking reality of which the patient may be fully aware, only dimly aware, or completely unaware. The anxiety-provoking reality may be an *intrapsychic* or *inner* reality (a prime example of which would be an affect — like anger or sadness) or an *interpersonal* or *outer* reality (something "real" about an object, the knowledge of which makes the patient anxious — perhaps something that disappoints or something that challenges).

THE CONCEPT OF RESISTANCE

Inner realities defended against include (1) anxiety-provoking impulses, (2) uncomfortable affects, and (3) distressing memories. Outer realities defended against include (1) acknowledging the reality of just how bad the infantile object really was and (2) recognizing that the transference object is neither as good as the patient had hoped (which disappoints the patient) nor as bad as the patient had feared (which challenges the patient's characteristic ways of experiencing his objects).

WHAT EASES ANXIETY?

The thing doing the defending may be simply one of the many ways the ego protects itself against anxiety (an ego defense). In other words, the defense that the ego mobilizes may be one of the well-known mechanisms of defense, like isolation of affect, repression, reaction formation, intellectualization, rationalization, or, more generally, a defense like the need to stay in control, the need to be self-sufficient, the need to be good, or the need to pretend that all is well.

But I am now suggesting that in addition to the more familiar intrapsychic defenses, there are also defenses that the ego/self mobilizes in order to protect itself against knowing the truth about its objects. Because of his need not to know, the patient clings to both his illusions and his distortions.

I am proposing, therefore, that we think of defenses (whether intrapsychic or interpersonal) as serving to protect the ego/self against the experience of anxiety-provoking realities. Whether the protection is of the ego against an anxiety-provoking inner reality or of the self against an anxiety-provoking outer reality, the defense serves to protect the individual against the experience of anxiety and/or pain.

IS THE DISTINCTION BETWEEN INTRAPSYCHIC AND INTERPERSONAL CLINICALLY USEFUL?

I believe that the intrapsychic realities against which the patient defends himself (for example, anger as a derivative of aggression) relate ultimately to the patient's objects; in other words, the anger, disappointment, frustration, or love that the patient experiences is always in relation to an external object and is not just a drive derivative.

I wanted to acknowledge, at least in theory, the presence of both anxiety-provoking intrapsychic realities (the province of classical psychoanalysis—a one-person model of the mind) and anxiety-provoking interpersonal realities (the province of self psychology and object relations theory—two-person models of the mind). But it is more useful, in the clinical situation, to ignore the distinction between the two different kinds of anxiety-provoking realities and to consider them, in actual practice, as one.

HOW DOES CONFLICT RELATE TO REALITY AND DEFENSE?

Ultimately, the tension within the patient, then, is between reality and defense. More accurately, perhaps, the tension is between an anxiety-provoking reality (whatever the degree of knowledge the patient has of it) and an anxiety-assuaging defense (which determines the patient's experience of that reality).

Alternatively, the tension within the patient is between his knowledge of reality and his experience of it, the latter a defense against the former.

We are saying, then, that there is ever tension within the patient between his capacity to know and his need not to know. From this it follows that anything serving to protect the patient against knowing constitutes a defense; the patient defends himself against facing anxiety-provoking realities by holding fast to anxiety-assuaging defenses.

WHAT IS THE RELATIONSHIP BETWEEN DEFENSE AND RESISTANCE?

The patient's defenses, in essence, constitute his resistance. In other words, anything that serves to protect the patient (whether the ego or the self) against the experience of anxiety and/or pain fuels the patient's resistance—and must ultimately be worked through before the patient can find his way to health.

The patient's need to deny his anger, his need to be angry instead of sad, his need to be depressed (in order not to feel, more acutely, his actual pain), his need to speak in a monotone, his need to keep the therapist at bay, his need to be always in control, his need to be confused (in order not to know)—all speak to the patient's defensive need to protect himself against anxiety and/or pain. All speak, therefore, to his resistance.

Similarly, the patient's reluctance to speak of his childhood, his reluctance to speak of the therapist, his lack of interest in understanding his internal process, his need to experience the therapist as the good parent he never had, his refusal to acknowledge just how disappointed he really is in his objects (past and present), his need to experience the therapist as the bad parent he did have—all speak to the patient's defensive need not to know. All speak, therefore, to his resistance.

WHAT IS THE DIFFERENCE BETWEEN TOXIC AND NONTOXIC REALITY?

I would suggest that the reality against which the patient as a child (in relation to the parent) defended himself may well have been a toxic reality, whereas the reality against which the patient now (in relation to the therapist) defends himself may well be a nontoxic reality. In both situations, however, the person defends himself against acknowledging that reality because it hurts too much to know the truth, whether about the infantile object or the transference object.

What is the toxic reality? The parent did not love the child as he should have been loved; but the child cannot possibly confront the pain of that. And so he takes the burden of the parent's badness upon himself (deciding that it must be he who is unlovable rather than his parent who is unloving) in order not to have to feel his devastation and his outrage. It is easier to experience himself as bad, his parent as good, than to acknowledge the horrid, toxic truth about just how unloving his parent really is.

To subsequent relationships, including, of course, the relationship with his therapist, the person brings both his wish for the good parent he never had and his fear that he will instead encounter the bad parent he did have.

What about the nontoxic realities? Ultimately the therapist is neither as good as the patient had hoped nor as bad as the patient had feared; but the patient does not want to accept the truth of that. And so he clings to his unrealistically positive misperceptions of the therapist—his illusions—in order not to have to face the pain of his disillusionment. And he clings to his unrealistically negative misperceptions of the therapist—his distortions—in order not to have to confront the reality that it could be, and could therefore have been, different.

The patient desperately needs to believe that the therapist will turn out to be the good parent he never had. It breaks his heart when he discovers that the therapist is not as good as he had hoped the therapist would be.

That the therapist is not as good as the patient would have wanted him to be is what I am here referring to as a nontoxic reality—and the patient's need is to deny this truth about his therapist, to deny his disenchantment.

On some level, the patient also needs to believe that the therapist will turn out to be as bad as the parent actually was. It makes him anxious to discover that the therapist is not as bad as he had assumed the therapist would be—assumptions based upon negative experiences he, the patient, had early on in relation to the toxic parent. Once the patient comes to know that it could have been otherwise with his parent, it is then that his heart breaks.

That the therapist is not as bad as the patient had expected him to be is, therefore, another nontoxic reality—and the patient's need (here too) is to deny this truth about his therapist, to deny this challenging of his reality.

And so there are toxic realities, against which the patient must defend himself because he cannot bear the pain of just how horrid his parent really was, and there are nontoxic realities, against which the patient tries to protect himself as well, because they challenge his ways of experiencing his objects, they challenge his need to experience his objects as other than who they are.

It is important, therefore, that we as therapists recognize and appreciate not only the patient's need to defend himself against acknowledging the horrid truth about his parent but also his need to defend himself against acknowledging the not-always-so-horrid truth about who we are, namely, that we are neither as good as he would have hoped nor as bad as he had feared. The truth about his parent is a toxic reality; the truth about us is a nontoxic reality—but the patient feels the need to defend himself against both. Both, therefore, constitute aspects of the resistance.

WHAT, THEN, IS THE RESISTANCE?

In sum, the resistance is made up of all those resistive forces that oppose the work of the treatment. On the one hand is the work to be done; on the other hand is the patient's opposition to doing that work. The conflicted patient is a defended patient is a resistant patient.

We can think, then, of the resistance (as it gets played out in the treatment situation) as speaking to all those resistive forces within the patient that interfere with the analytic process, all those resistive forces that impede the patient's progress in the treatment, all those resistive forces that oppose the patient's movement toward health.

Perhaps we could even say, with respect to the resistance, that one resists feeling what he knows he should feel and resists doing what he knows he should do.

TWO

Resistance as Failure to Grieve

> **WHAT DOES THE CHILD DO WHEN FACED WITH THE UNBEARABLY PAINFUL REALITY OF THE PARENTAL LIMITATIONS?**

The child, when confronted with the excruciatingly painful reality of just how disappointing his parent really is, cannot possibly come to terms with it. Instead, he defends himself against the pain of his heartache by taking upon himself the burden of the parent's badness (thereby creating a distorted sense of himself as bad). By so doing, he is able to preserve the relationship with the parent—uncontaminated by his rageful disappointment—and his illusions about the parent as good.

Feeling bad about himself seems like a small price to pay as long as it enables him to maintain his belief in the parent's goodness, his hope that perhaps someday, somehow, someway, if he can but get it right, his parent's love will be forthcoming.

HOW DOES INTERNALIZING THE PARENTAL BADNESS APPLY TO SURVIVORS OF ABUSE?

Taking on the badness as his own (in order to defend himself against acknowledging the reality of that badness in the parent) is something that happens all the time with survivors of childhood abuse.

It is easier for the abused child to experience himself as having deserved the abuse than to accept the reality of just how abusive the parent really was, easier to fault himself and feel guilt than to fault the parent and feel anger. In other words, it is easier to experience himself as bad than to confront the reality of the parent's badness.

By sacrificing himself, the child can deny the parental badness and can cling to the hope that if he tries really hard to be really good, then he may yet be able to get his parent (or someone who is a stand-in for his parent) to love him as he wants to be—and should have been—loved. After all, if the badness resides within himself, then he has more control over it than if it resides within the parent.

And so the child holds on to the illusion that his parent was good and to the distortion that it was he who was (and is) bad, although the reality is that it is he who was (and is) good and the parent who was bad.

HOW DO EARLY-ON TOXIC FAILURES CREATE THE NEED FOR ILLUSION AND DISTORTION?

Had the child been able to face just how limited the parent really was and had he been able to master his disappointment and his outrage, then he would have had neither the need to cling to the illusion of the parent as good nor the need to take the burden of the parent's badness upon himself. Illusion is the result of that denial; distortion is the result of that internalization. Both illusion and distortion (with respect to the self and, by way of projection, the object) become part of the way the patient experiences his world.

In other words, had the child been able to confront the intolerably painful reality of just how bad the toxic parent really was, then he would not now have the need for either illusion or distortion.

Illusions and distortions arise, therefore, in the context of the patient's inability to confront the early-on parental failures and grieve them. The presence of illusion and distortion speaks to ungrieved losses.

WHAT IS THE RELATIONSHIP, THEN, BETWEEN THE FAILURE TO GRIEVE AND THE NEED FOR DEFENSE?

The presence of illusion and distortion speaks to the patient's failure to grieve. The illusions and distortions arose, originally, in the context of defending the child against confronting the horrid reality of just how bad things were. They serve, in the here and now, to defend the patient against confronting the not-always-so-horrid-but-nonetheless-anxiety-provoking reality of things as they are — namely, that they are neither as good as he had hoped they would be (which disappoints) nor as bad as he had feared they would be (which challenges).

As long as the patient clings to his illusions, hoping against hope that his objects will change, and as long as he clings to his distortions, ever expecting now to be failed as he was once failed, then the patient has not yet done all the grieving he will eventually have to do in order to extricate himself from the past and from his compulsive need to recreate that past in the present.

The presence of defense speaks, then, to the patient's failure to grieve. And from this it follows that the patient's resistance is fueled by his refusal to grieve.

WHAT DO WE MEAN BY THE REPETITION COMPULSION?

St. Paul could have been speaking about the repetition compulsion when he said: "The good that I know I should do, I don't; and the bad that I know I shouldn't do, I do." Equally compellingly, Paul Russell (1980) has suggested that people, under the sway of the repetition compulsion, find themselves repeating what they would rather not.

Both descriptions capture the essence of just how powerful, just how insidious, just how sabotaging, and just how relentless our unconscious repetitions can actually be.

HOW DOES IT COME TO PASS THAT THE REPETITION COMPULSION HAS SUCH A PROFOUND IMPACT ON WHAT WE FEEL AND DO?

The person who has not yet been able to confront, head on, his pain about the parental limitations and has therefore not yet grieved brings to subsequent relationships both his illusions and his distortions, both his unrealistically positive perceptions about his objects and his unrealistically negative perceptions about himself and, by way of projection, his objects.

Under the sway of the repetition compulsion, the patient delivers his pathology (both his wish for good and his fear of bad) into the transference — in the form of his illusions and his distortions. The patient finds himself longing for the therapist to be good (what we refer to as the patient's relentless pursuit of infantile gratification in the transference), even as he is afraid that the therapist will be bad, afraid that the therapist will confirm his worst suspicions (what we refer to as the patient's compulsive reenactments of his internal dramas in the transference).

Paradoxically, even as he hopes for the best, he fears the worst. Even as he longs for the therapist to be good and to make up the difference to him, he needs the therapist to be bad, in order to confirm his worst fears — because that is all he has ever known and all he is familiar with.

> ## HOW DOES THE REPETITION COMPULSION RELATE TO THE WISH FOR CONTAINMENT?

Russell (1982) goes on to suggest that in the repetition is a healthy wish for containment. Intrinsic to the patient's relentless pursuit of infantile gratification and intrinsic to his compulsive reenactments of his internal dramas is a wish to be contained.

We say of the repetition compulsion, therefore, that it always has both an unhealthy aspect and a healthy aspect. The repetition compulsion is powered by the unhealthy need to keep things exactly as they have always been, a neurotic compulsion to repeat what is known, even if pathological. At the same time, the repetition compulsion is fueled by the healthy need to have, first, more of same and then something different, a healthy need to recreate in the here and now the original traumatic failure situation in the hope that perhaps this time the outcome will be better.

There is, then, a constant re-creating of the past in the present. The neurotic part of the patient is invested in keeping things the same. The neurotic compulsion to preserve the old in the new is the patient's way of remaining loyal, even after all these years, to his infantile object. The past is, after all, the only thing he has ever known; it's familiar, it's comfortable, and it's safe.

But the healthy part of the patient wants the resolution, this time, to be different, and so the compulsion to repeat is also powered by the healthy urge to turn passive to active, the healthy urge to transform an experience passively endured into a situation actively created. The wish is for belated mastery; the wish is to be able, at last, to create a different outcome.

> ## HOW DOES THE REPETITION COMPULSION BOTH HINDER AND HELP?

That the patient compulsively repeats his past in the present is, therefore, double-edged. On the one hand, the compulsive repetitions fuel the transference, fuel the resistance—and therefore impede the patient's progress in the treatment. On the other hand, it is by way of working through the transference, by way of overcoming the resistance, that the patient is able, at last, to achieve belated mastery of the early-on environmental failures by doing now what he could not possibly do as a child—grieve.

HOW DOES THE TREATMENT SITUATION CREATE THE OPPORTUNITY TO GRIEVE?

The treatment situation offers the patient an opportunity to confront the intolerably painful reality of just how bad the parent really was and how deeply scarred the patient is now as a result of that. Within the context of the safety provided by the relationship with his therapist, the patient is able, finally, to feel the pain against which he has spent a lifetime defending himself.

WHAT IS THE RELATIONSHIP BETWEEN GRIEVING AND THE REPETITION COMPULSION?

In grieving, one relinquishes the need for the repetition compulsion (Russell 1982). We repeat in order not to have to feel the pain of our disappointment. As we confront our pain, as we confront at last the unbearably painful toxic realities of the early-on parental failures, we no longer have the same need to repeat (the old in the new). In grieving, we let go of those unconscious repetitions that have obstructed our movement forward.

WHAT DOES IT MEAN TO GRIEVE?

As part of the grieving he must do, the patient must come to accept the fact that he is ultimately powerless to do anything to make his objects, both past and present, different. (He can and should do things to change himself, but he cannot change his objects—and he will have to come to terms with that.) He must feel, to the very depths of his soul, his anguish and his outrage that his parent was as he was, his therapist is as he is, and the world is as it is. Such is the work of grieving.

Genuine grief involves confronting the reality of how it really was and is. It means accepting those realities, knowing that there is nothing that he can now do to make them any different. It means coming to terms with the fact that neither he himself nor the objects in his world will ever be exactly as he would have wanted them to be.

Grieving means knowing that he may well be psychically scarred in the here and now because of things that happened early on but that he must live with that, knowing that there is nothing that can now be done to undo the original damage. Perhaps there are ways to compensate for the childhood injuries, but there is no way to undo them and certainly no way to extract from his objects in the here and now recompense for the wounds sustained early on.

Genuine grief means being able to sit with the horror of it all, the outrage, the pain, the despair, the hurt, the sense of betrayal, the woundedness; it means accepting one's ultimate powerlessness in the face of all this; and it means deciding to move on as best one can with what one has—sadder perhaps, but wiser too.

WHAT IS PSEUDO-GRIEF?

Grieving does not mean being depressed, feeling sorry for oneself, blaming oneself, blaming others, or feeling victimized. The patient who faults, blames, and accuses is not accepting the reality of things as they are. Nor is the patient who protests that it isn't fair, that he is entitled to more. Nor is the patient who insists that his objects change, demands that his objects be other than who they are.

Such patients are not accepting reality; they are refusing to accept it. They are not confronting reality and doing what they must do to come to terms with it; instead, they are refusing to confront reality, they are refusing to grieve. They are doing something that I refer to as pseudo-grief, a display of emotion that mimics grief but is not the real thing. Pseudo-grief is used to defend against honest grief.

A Hasidic saying (Buber 1966) speaks to this distinction: "There are two kinds of sorrow. . . . When a man broods over the misfortunes that have come upon him, when he cowers in a corner and despairs of help—that is a bad kind of sorrow. . . . The other kind is the honest grief of a man whose house has burned down, who feels his need deep in his soul and begins to build anew" (p. 231). The bad kind of sorrow is what I am here describing as pseudo-grief; it speaks to a man's refusal to confront reality. The heartfelt grief of a man who has confronted his pain and feels it deeply is the response of a healthy man who does not need to defend against loss.

HOW DOES THE PATIENT'S EXPERIENCE OF INTERNAL IMPOVERISHMENT SPEAK TO HIS FAILURE TO GRIEVE?

Imagine the following scenario: The patient, in treatment for many years now, has made significant improvements in the external circumstances of his life but still speaks of a profound loneliness and a relentless despair. He is deeply attached to his therapist and feels held by him in the sessions, but between sessions he cannot sustain any of those good feelings and instead feels desperately alone and empty.

The patient's internal impoverishment, the paucity of healthy psychic structure, is the price he has paid for his unwillingness (perhaps inability) to grieve his past. It is the price he pays for his refusal to face the reality of just how bad it really was.

Because the patient has never made his peace with just how limited his parent really was, he has a distorted sense of himself (as limited, as incapable, as having been so damaged from way back that he is not now able to do anything on his own to ease his pain), underlying illusions (that his contemporary objects and, in particular, his therapist will be able to ease his pain), and deep entitlement (a profound conviction that this is his due).

WHAT IS THE REFRAIN OF THE PATIENT WITH UNMOURNED LOSSES?

It is as if the patient is saying, "I can't, you can, and you should." As long as he clings to his distortions (I can't), his illusions (you can), and his entitlement (you should), his forward movement will be impeded.

WHAT IS INVOLVED IN THERAPEUTIC IMPASSES?

The patient will not get better as long as he clings, usually unconsciously, to those distortions, those illusions, and that entitlement.

As long as the patient refuses to grieve, refuses to remember, refuses to relive, refuses to let himself really feel, in his gut, the depths of his devastation and his outrage about just how bad it really was, then he will be destined to be forever misunderstanding his present in terms of his unresolved past.

Therapeutic impasses arise in the context of the patient's refusal to grieve and his reluctance to let go of his sense of himself as damaged and incapable, his sense of the therapist as able but unwilling, and his sense of himself as wrongfully deprived and therefore entitled now to recompense.

As Sheldon Kopp (1969) observes:

> The adult in whom the unmet, unmourned child dwells, stubbornly insists that he has the power to make someone love him, or else to make them feel sorry for not doing so. Appeasing, wheedling, bribing, or bullying are carried out in stubborn hope that if only he is submissive enough, sneaky enough, bad enough, upset enough, something enough . . . then he will get his own way. [p. 31]

Therapeutic impasses speak to the patient's refusal to confront the reality that it is ultimately his responsibility to do with his life what he will. Admittedly, it was not his fault then, but it is his responsibility now.

As long as the patient locates the responsibility for change within others (and not within himself), as long as he experiences the locus of control as external (and not internal), then his experience of his objects will be one of bitter disappointment, angry dissatisfaction, and painful defeat — and he will be ever yearning for things to be other than how they really are.

MORE GENERALLY, HOW DOES THE PATIENT'S FAILURE TO GRIEVE RELATE TO THE RESISTANCE?

As long as the patient refuses to confront certain intolerably painful early-on realities and buries his pain, then he will be destined to be forever recreating the past in the present. Because of childhood losses never properly mourned, he will find himself in the treatment situation both desperately yearning for the good parent he never had and compulsively recapitulating with the therapist the early-on traumatic failure situation.

In other words, because of his failure to grieve, he will be relentless in his pursuit of infantile gratification (which will fuel the positive transference) and compulsive in his reenactment of his unresolved childhood dramas (which will fuel the negative transference).

As long as he refuses to grieve, the patient will remain stuck in the treatment and in his life.

THREE

Mastering Resistance by Way of Grieving

WHAT MUST THE PATIENT COME TO UNDERSTAND BEFORE HE CAN MOVE ON?

If the patient is to be able to move forward in the treatment and in his life, he must come to understand that his therapist will not be able to make him all better, will not be able to fill him up inside, and will not be able to make up the difference to him and make right the wrongs done, much as both patient and therapist might have wished this to be possible.

Eventually the patient must feel his disappointment, his heartache, and his outrage about all this; he must face, head on, the intolerably painful reality of the therapist's limitations—namely, the therapist's inability to make up entirely for the bad parenting the patient had as a child.

WHAT IS THE ROLE OF GRIEVING WITH RESPECT TO THE EARLY-ON PARENTAL FAILURES?

Ultimately, the work the patient must do with respect to the resistance is grief work. Instead of denying the reality of the parent's very real shortcomings and inadequacies, the patient needs to be able to face that reality head on. Instead of experiencing the badness as residing within himself, he must be able to recognize that it is the parent who was limited. Instead of hating himself, he must be able to rage at the disappointing parent. It was not the patient who was unworthy and undeserving; it was his parent who was lacking. Instead of clinging to the illusion that he may someday be able to extract the goodies from his parent (or a stand-in for his parent), he must be able to accept the fact of his utter powerlessness to make his objects change.

Once the patient begins to confront the reality of just how limited the parent really was and how great a price the patient has paid for those limitations, once he begins to face the unbearable pain of his disappointment that things were as they were, and once he finally gains access to his long-repressed outrage and sorrow, then the patient will be able to relinquish the distortions, illusions, and entitlement around which he has organized himself and his experience of the world.

It will be as the patient grieves that he will master his resistance.

WHAT IS THE RELATIONSHIP BETWEEN GRIEVING AND INTERNALIZING?

It is only as the patient grieves the reality of what the parent did not give him that he can begin to appreciate and to take in all those things that the parent did give him. As Kopp (1969) writes: "By no longer refusing to mourn the loss of the parents whom he wished for but never had, he can get to keep whatever was really there for him" (p. 33).

So, too, with respect to the therapist. It will be only as the patient confronts the reality of what the therapist does not give him, and comes to terms with that, that he will be able to appreciate and to take in all those things that the therapist does give him.

HOW DOES WORKING THROUGH THE TRANSFERENCE INVOLVE RELINQUISHING THE DEFENSES?

The therapeutic work requires of the patient that he make his peace with the fact that the therapist is neither as good as he had hoped nor as bad as he had feared. The patient makes his peace with the discrepancy between what he comes to know as real and what he had imagined was real by way of working through the transference, both the disrupted positive transference and the negative transference.

Working through the transference is the process by which the patient is enabled, gradually, to let go of the illusions and distortions to which he has spent a lifetime clinging in order not to have to know the truth about his objects, both infantile and contemporary. As the patient's illusions and distortions are relinquished, the patient's (defensive) need for his objects to be other than who they are becomes transformed into a capacity to experience, and to accept, them as they are.

HOW IS PARADOX INVOLVED?

Paradoxically, working through the transference is the process by which need is transformed into capacity (to tolerate reality as it is); but it is the presence of that capacity that facilitates the ultimate working through of the transference.

HOW DOES WORKING THROUGH THE TRANSFERENCE INVOLVE GRIEVING?

Need is transformed into capacity by way of resolving the transference — a working-through process that involves confronting certain realities (both the toxic reality of the infantile object and the nontoxic reality of the transference object) and grieving them.

As the unhealthy resistive forces that impede the patient's progress are gradually worked through and transformed, the healthy forces that urge the patient forward will be given free rein and the patient will move toward health.

> ## HOW DOES RESOLVING THE TRANSFERENCE PROMOTE THE PATIENT'S MENTAL HEALTH?

As we discussed earlier, mental health has to do with the capacity to experience reality as it is; mental illness (pathology) has to do with the need to experience it as it is not, in ways contaminated by the past.

To the extent that the patient holds fast to his illusions and distortions and refuses to face reality, to that extent will the patient be described as resistant. But to the extent that the patient is able to experience reality as it is and to grieve past and present heartbreakingly painful realities, to that extent will the patient get better.

When the patient has overcome his transferential need to experience reality as it is not and is able to tolerate reality as it is, we speak of the resistance as having been mastered.

FOUR

Grieving, Internalization, and Development of Capacity

WHAT IS SELF PSYCHOLOGY?

In its barest bones, self psychology is a theory about grieving, grieving the loss of illusions—illusions about the perfection (or the perfectibility) of the self and/or the object.

Self psychology is about illusion (the need for illusion) and disillusionment (working through or grieving the loss of illusion); it's about having illusions, losing them, and recovering from their loss.

As part of the grieving process, the functions performed by the disillusioning object are internalized and laid down as structure—structure that transforms the patient's narcissistic need for perfection into a capacity to tolerate imperfection, structure that transforms the patient's need for external regulation of his self-esteem into a capacity to provide such regulation internally.

In summary, self psychology is about transforming need (the

need for external reinforcement, the need for illusion, the need for perfection) into capacity (the capacity to accept the object as it is); it's about internalizing functions, modifying need, mapping out structure, developing capacity, filling in deficit, and consolidating the self.

HOW DOES SELF PSYCHOLOGY CONCEIVE OF THE RELATIONSHIP BETWEEN GRIEVING, INTERNALIZATION, AND STRUCTURALIZATION?

It is to self psychology that we will look in order to enhance our understanding of the relationship between grieving and internalizing the good.

The self psychologists have conceptualized a model for development of self structure in which empathic failure provides an opportunity for structural growth. More specifically, self psychology informs us that it is the experience of properly grieved frustration, against a backdrop of gratification, that provides the impetus for internalization and the laying down of structure.

With respect to the child: When the parent has been good and is then bad, the child masters his disappointment in the frustrating parent by internalizing the good that had been there prior to the introduction of the bad. He defensively and adaptively takes in the good parent as part of the grieving process, so that he can preserve internally a piece of the original experience of external goodness.

Note that, according to self theory, good gets inside as a result not of experiencing gratification but of working through frustration against a backdrop of gratification. In other words, self structure develops as a result not of the experience of an empathically responsive parent but of working through disappointment in an otherwise empathically responsive parent, working through a disrupted positive (narcissistic) transference.

In other words, the impetus for internalization is the failure itself. As long as the child is having his needs met, there is no impetus for internalization because there is nothing that needs to be mastered. It is only with the experience that things are not always as the child would have wanted them to be, that there is incentive for the child to make internal what had once been reliably present externally.

And so it is that empathic failure, against a backdrop of empathic responsiveness, can be the occasion for the accretion of internal structure. Self psychology refers to such a process of growth as transmuting internalization by way of optimal disillusionment — in other words, the building of self structure by way of working through, or grieving, the loss of illusion.

HOW DOES THE PATIENT BECOME AUTONOMOUS?

Heinz Hartmann (1939) conceived of internalization as a process whereby external regulatory functions (provided by the environment) are gradually replaced by internal regulatory functions (provided by the self) — such that the self becomes autonomous, independent of its objects.

The self psychologists incorporated Hartmann's ideas into their conceptualization of transmuting internalization as that process whereby the patient makes internal those selfobject functions that had once been external, a transformative process that enables the patient to do for himself what he had once needed from his objects. As the patient develops the capacity to provide for himself, it becomes easier to tolerate the reality that his objects will not always be as good or as perfect as he would have wanted them to be.

In other words, the patient's need for a good (perfect) parent becomes transformed into a capacity to be for himself the good parent he never had. And although he never gives up entirely his need for selfobjects (to fill in for those parts of himself that are absent or impaired), he becomes better able to tolerate the separate existence of objects, with their own identities and their own centers of initiative.

WHAT IS THE DISTINCTION BETWEEN NONTRAUMATIC (OR OPTIMAL) AND TRAUMATIC DISILLUSIONMENT?

Self psychology suggests that we think of a disillusionment (a frustration, disappointment, or loss) as nontraumatic if and only if it can be processed and worked through, that is, grieved. By the same token, a disillusionment is traumatic if and only if it cannot, for whatever the reason, be mastered.

Let us imagine that a therapist has just informed his patient that he will be away for four weeks in August. Will this be a nontraumatic or a traumatic loss for the patient?

The answer, of course, is that it depends. If the patient is eventually able to master his disappointment, then, by definition, the failure will have been a nontraumatic (or an optimal) one. If, on the other hand, the patient is never able to master his disappointment, then the failure will have been a traumatic one.

Nontraumatic disappointments, then, are losses properly grieved; traumatic disappointments are losses improperly grieved.

WHY IS THE DISTINCTION BETWEEN NONTRAUMATIC AND TRAUMATIC SO CRUCIAL?

I will later be developing the idea that nontraumatic frustration provides the impetus for internalizing one kind of object, namely, the good object, whereas traumatic frustration provides the impetus for internalizing another kind of object, namely, the bad object.

In other words, nontraumatic frustration results in healthy development (healthy structure) and traumatic frustration results in pathological development (pathogenic structure).

HOW DOES SELF PSYCHOLOGY INFORM OUR UNDERSTANDING OF THE DEVELOPMENT OF HEALTHY STRUCTURE?

In order to understand how it is that new good structure is added, we look to self psychology, which spells out beautifully the relationship between working through, or grieving, the loss of transference illusions and the laying down of healthy structure. From self theory, we know that optimal disillusionment is the process by which transmuting internalization and structural growth occur.

I believe that self psychology provides a more comprehensive model for understanding psychic growth than does either classical psychoanalysis or object relations theory.

My claim will be that there are some important parallels to be drawn between the laying down of self structure (the province of self theory) and the laying down of drive structure (the province of drive theory).

Before we pursue this further, let us first understand what we actually mean by structure and the development of capacity.

WHAT IS MEANT BY PSYCHIC STRUCTURE (OR CAPACITY)?

Psychic structures are configurations in the mind that are relatively enduring over time, relatively resistant to change, and, most importantly, perform functions.

The drive structures of classical psychoanalysis (the drive-regulating introjects in the ego and superego) perform the function of drive regulation (that is, drive modulation or control). In fact, classical psychoanalysis is about development of the ego and superego (or conscience) from the id. It is about transformation of id energy into ego and superego structure, transformation of the need for external drive control into the capacity to provide such control internally.

The self structures of self psychology—the ambitions and purposes of the ego, the goals and aspirations of the ego ideal—perform the function of self-esteem regulation (or, as it is more commonly called, self regulation). Not surprisingly, self psychology is about development of the self—more specifically, the ego and ego ideal. It is about transformation of narcissistic energy into ego and ego ideal structure, transformation of the need for external reinforcement of the self-esteem into the capacity to provide such reinforcement internally.

Structures (whether drive structures or self structures) perform functions that enable capacity.

HOW DOES SELF PSYCHOLOGY INFORM OUR UNDERSTANDING OF THE PROCESS BY WHICH INTERNAL DRIVE REGULATION DEVELOPS?

As we know, the province of drive theorists is development of the ego and superego proper (or conscience); their focus is on the id drives and the regulation (or control) of those drives. Initially, according to drive theory, the child's libidinal and aggressive drives are said to be regulated externally by the infantile drive object. In other words, some drives are gratified and some are frustrated.

Over the course of development, the function of drive regulation is internalized, and regulatory structures develop in both the ego and superego. Such structures are drive regulators, drive-regulating introjects; these introjects have taken over the function of drive regulation once performed by the drive object.

Classical psychoanalysis, then, is really all about transformation of the drives into drive-regulating structures in the ego and superego. As energy is transformed into structure, need is transformed into capacity: the need for external drive regulation is replaced by the capacity for internal drive regulation.

HOW DO WE DESCRIBE SUCH A TRANSFORMATIVE PROCESS?

We can express such a process of transformation in a number of ways. We speak about transformation of the need for immediate gratification into the capacity to tolerate delay or the need for absolute gratification into the capacity to derive pleasure from relative gratification. More generally, we speak of transforming the need for external regulation of the libidinal and aggressive drives into a capacity to regulate such drives internally.

HOW ARE ANAL STRIVINGS TRANSFORMED INTO HEALTHY CAPACITY?

Let us consider the following scenario: The mother of a 2-year-old boy tells him to put his toys away, to keep his trucks and cars in the playroom, not to stick his fingers in electrical outlets, not to hit his little sister or throw her out the window, not to mess with his food, not to pull the cat's tail, and so on. The mother is telling her son what he should and shouldn't do; in essence, she is telling him which ones of his aggressive impulses can be gratified, which ones cannot.

The child comes to understand that to comply is to get mother's approval and to defy is to get her disapproval.

So the child learns to be good, to comply, to modulate his aggressive impulses when mother is around and, in time, to modulate them even when mother is not around.

The mother's prescriptions and proscriptions (her shoulds and shouldn'ts) become internalized in the form of superego dictates, which then regulate, internally, the expression of the child's aggressive strivings.

And so it is that the superego begins to develop.

But now let's consider another scenario. The little 2-year-old boy is trying to put his toys away because his mother has asked him to, but he's having some trouble getting all the toys back in the box.

A sensitive mother will recognize the child's plight. He wants to be able to comply, he wants to be good, but he does not yet have the capacity to do what he has been told to do; he does not yet have the skills to implement his wish. Mother, appreciating this, does not put extra pressure on him; instead, she encourages him to take his time and to do it slowly, one toy at a time. She may even sit down on the floor beside him in order to demonstrate to him how this can be done.

And if the child is beginning to fret or have a temper tantrum, she handles it by holding him, providing her calmness to soothe him, so that he can recover control.

In essence, she is demonstrating how aggressive impulses can be controlled and regulated; she is offering the child's ego a model for executing its function of drive regulation, drive modulation, drive control. The mother's demonstration of how the child can regulate his aggressive drives gets internalized in the form of internal ego controls and becomes part of the drive-regulating matrix of the ego.

And so it is that the ego develops.

In summary, the mother's reactions to the child's expression of his aggressive impulses get taken into the superego in the form of drive-regulating introjects. But the mother's demonstration of reality-based, adaptive ways of controlling aggressive impulses provides role modeling, which the child can internalize in the form of ego introjects (or identifications).

In other words, if the parent has functioned as a reasonably gratifying and only optimally frustrating regulator of the child's anal strivings to oppose, to thwart, and to challenge, then the child is able, step by step, bit by bit, to internalize the drive-regulating functions performed by the parent and to develop internal controls where before he had needed to rely upon the parent for external control. As ego and superego structure develops, need is transformed into capacity; the destructive need to discharge aggressive energy almost indiscriminately is transformed into the capacity to be healthily self-assertive and to direct one's aggressive energy into constructive channels.

HOW ARE OEDIPAL STRIVINGS TRANSFORMED INTO HEALTHY CAPACITY?

Let us think about a little 3-year-old girl's oedipal strivings, her (usually unconscious) urge to have sex with her father and to triumph over her mother. If all goes well, such needs become tamed over time and transformed into capacity. In other words, if the little girl's oedipal strivings are gently but firmly frustrated — that is, benevolently contained by an optimally frustrating parent — and if the little girl has the opportunity to process and master such frustration, then her incestuous and matricidal impulses become transformed bit by bit into the capacity to take initiative in the pursuit of her dreams without the burden of guilt.

MORE GENERALLY, WHAT IS THE RESULT OF TAMING ID NEEDS?

Where once there was energy, now there is structure. Where once there was need, now there is capacity; where once need for external regulation of the drives, now the capacity for internal regulation of them. The acquisition of such capacity makes external regulation unnecessary.

HOW DOES SELF PSYCHOLOGY INFORM OUR UNDERSTANDING OF THE PROCESS BY WHICH INTERNAL SELF REGULATION DEVELOPS?

Let us now shift from drive theory to self theory, where the emphasis is upon development of the self and the focus is upon the self-esteem and its regulation. Initially, according to self theory, the child's self-esteem is regulated externally by the infantile selfobject. Over the course of development, the function of self-esteem regulation is internalized, and regulatory structures develop in both the ego and ego ideal.

Heinz Kohut (1966) suggests that there are basically two narcissistic lines of development: one involves transformation of the grandiose self into the ambitions and purposes of the ego; the other involves transformation of the idealized selfobject into the goals and aspirations of the ego ideal.

In essence, one line of development involves transformation of the perfect self (or, more accurately, the need for a perfect self) into ambition. The other line involves transformation of the perfect selfobject (or, more accurately, the need for a perfect selfobject) into goals.

WHAT IS THE RELATIONSHIP BETWEEN SUCH TRANSFORMATIONS AND WORKING THROUGH THE TRANSFERENCE?

These transformations are the result of working through disruptions of the positive (narcissistic) transference—namely, working through optimal disillusionment. The disillusionment is with the object, not the self. It is with the selfobject, be it the mirroring selfobject that disappoints by failing to provide mirroring confirmation of the self's perfection or the idealized selfobject that disappoints by turning out to be less than perfect.

Working through disillusionment with the selfobject results, ultimately, in development of the capacity to tolerate imperfection in the self (the first line of development) and development of the capacity to tolerate imperfection in the object (the second line of development).

WHAT HAPPENS TO THE NEED FOR A PERFECT SELF?

With respect to the first line of narcissistic development: Think about the infant's need for perfection of the self and mirroring confirmation of that perfection by the mirroring selfobject.

Consider the mother who looks on with delight and admiration as her little baby plays in his crib with his rattle, trying as best he can to achieve mastery of it. She thinks that he is the most beautiful and the smartest little baby in the world. Clearly she is performing as a mirroring selfobject and is deriving pleasure from her little baby and his attempts at mastery.

We can easily believe that this lucky little baby, as a grown-up, will have internalized his mother's admiring interest and will now be able to derive his own pleasure from his attempts at mastery. In essence, the child's need for perfection of the self and mirroring confirmation of that perfection by the object will have become transformed into a healthy capacity to direct his efforts toward mastery and to derive pleasure from his pursuits.

We can think of this first line of development, then, as involving transformation of "Look at me, mirror; I am perfect, am I not?" into "I may not be perfect, but I know I am good enough; I am able to apply myself to whatever task is at hand, and I derive pleasure from mastering challenges and overcoming obstacles."

We speak of the transformation of his narcissism in the sense that, whereas once he needed to see himself as perfect (and to have that perfection confirmed by others), he is now able to experience himself as imperfect but certainly plenty good enough.

WHAT HAPPENS TO THE NEED FOR A PERFECT OBJECT?

With respect to the second line of narcissistic development: Think about the child's need to be able to experience his parent as the embodiment of idealized perfection and then, through fantasized merger with the idealized object, to partake of its perfection, strength, and tranquillity. The function performed by the idealized selfobject is provision of an opportunity for the child to invest his objects with perfection so that he can look up to them for guidance and inspiration.

We can easily believe that this lucky little child, as a grown-up, will have internalized, in the form of his own standards of excellence, the qualities that the parent had embodied. In essence, the child's need for perfection of the selfobject will have become transformed into a healthy capacity to rely, for direction, upon his own internalized standards of excellence. No longer will he have the same need to idealize his objects.

Where once the child invested his parent with perfection so that he could look up to the parent for guidance and inspiration, now he has the capacity to provide such direction on his own. We can describe such a process as one that involves transformation of "I look at you and imagine that you are perfect; I too become perfect through my union with you" into "I now have my own goals and aspirations; I have my own dreams to pursue, my own potential to realize."

ARE THE INTERNALIZED STANDARDS REALISTIC OR PERFECTIONISTIC?

How do we characterize the goals that develop from working through disenchantment with the idealized selfobject?

In the self psychology literature, different answers have been suggested. Sometimes the goals are referred to as idealized, perfectionistic standards. At other times the goals are referred to, simply, as standards of excellence, implying a tamed perfection and easier attainability.

In fact, part of working through disappointment in the idealized selfobject involves letting go of the need for perfection in the object; it involves taming and modifying one's expectations of perfection. What gets internalized and integrated into the ego ideal is, therefore, a tamed and modified perfectionism, something less idealistic, more realistic, more attainable.

If the working-through process is not completed and the perfectionism is not tamed and modified, then the individual is destined always to be feeling chronically inadequate, defective, a failure — the plight of the narcissist.

WHAT ARE EMPTY DEPRESSIONS?

In fact, the empty depressions (the so-called narcissistic deficiency states) from which narcissistic personalities often suffer are the result of the (experienced) discrepancy between actual and wished for, the conflict between ego and ego ideal.

The patient who suffers from an empty depression has weak ambition and/or unachievable goals. If he has weak ambition (or an impaired drive for mastery), he will have difficulty harnessing his energy in order to spur himself onward. If he has unachievable goals, he will never be able to get there anyway (no matter how strong his ambition) — because it's an impossible journey.

The weaker the ambition and the more unrealistic the goal, the greater the discrepancy between what he will be able to do and what he would have wished to do.

The greater the discrepancy, the greater the sense of shame. The patient's experience will be of narcissistic mortification and humiliation because of his failure to fulfill his potential.

This conception of empty depression as a result of discrepancy between the ego ideal and the ego is, of course, very similar to Edward Bibring's (1953) conceptualization of depression as a result of tension between narcissistic aspirations and the ego's awareness of its failure to live up to such aspirations.

WHAT RESULTS FROM WORKING THROUGH DISRUPTED POSITIVE TRANSFERENCES?

As a result of working through disruptions of the positive (narcissistic) transference, the need for reinforcement by the mirroring selfobject will have become transformed into a capacity to motivate oneself and to derive pleasure from one's attempts at mastery, and the need for reinforcement by way of merger with the idealized selfobject will have become transformed into a capacity to have one's own vision about what is possible.

Whereas the first line of development (culminating in the achievement of healthy ambition) has to do with the means, the second line of development (culminating in the achievement of realizable goals) has to do with the ends.

Self psychology, then, informs us about transformation of the need for external reinforcement into the capacity to provide reinforcement internally.

WHAT IS THE RELATIONSHIP BETWEEN THE PATIENT'S NEED FOR PERFECTION AND, MORE GENERALLY, HIS NEED FOR ILLUSION?

Strictly speaking, self psychology is about the patient's need for perfection and his evolving capacity to tolerate imperfection. Our interest here, however, will be in what self psychology tells us about the process whereby need is transformed into capacity, more specifically, the patient's need for his objects to be other than (better than) they are becomes transformed into a capacity to accept them as they are—as the patient comes to terms with their limitations and his disenchantment with them.

As the patient grieves the loss of his illusions, he develops the capacity to accept what he cannot change and to direct himself toward changing what he can. As the patient works through disrupted positive (narcissistic) transference, he becomes able to sit with his disappointment and to overcome his need for illusion.

In other words, as the patient's need for the object to perform certain regulatory functions is transformed into the capacity to perform such functions on his own, there is no longer the same need for the object to fill in for missing psychic structure. As the need is diminished, there is a greater capacity to accept the object as it is.

WHAT DOES IT MEAN TO DEVELOP MATURE CAPACITY?

Whether we address ourselves to drive regulation or self regulation, the process of growth (both developmental and psychotherapeutic) is accompanied by the transformation of energy into structure, need into capacity.

But if we choose not to limit ourselves to considering the fate of untamed libidinal and aggressive drives or the fate of the narcissistic need for perfection, then we can think, more generally, of the process of growth from the point of view of transforming the infantile need to experience one's objects as other than who they are into a healthy capacity to experience them as they are.

Such a perspective, moving beyond the confines of drive theory and self theory, addresses itself to that difficult process by which the individual matures, gradually coming to terms with the painful reality that his objects will not always be exactly as he would have wanted them to be.

WHY DO WE TURN TO SELF THEORY TO INFORM OUR UNDERSTANDING OF THIS TRANSFORMATIVE PROCESS?

Although self theory is primarily interested in the forms and transformations of narcissism, it demonstrates so beautifully the process by which positive experiences are internally recorded and structuralized in the form of healthy capacity that we can use it to inform our understanding, more generally, of structural growth (whether of the child as he grows up or the patient as he heals).

Self psychology has an outstanding contribution to make to our understanding of how infantile need is transformed into mature capacity. It is therefore to self psychology, with its emphasis on illusion, disillusionment, grieving, internalization, and structure building that we will look in order to enhance our understanding of how the individual comes to need less and less for his objects to be a certain way and comes to appreciate more and more that they are as they are. It is this transformative process (of replacing need with capacity) that is the process whereby the resistance is gradually overcome and the individual moves forward.

FIVE

Development of Pathology

WHAT IS THE VILLAIN IN THIS PIECE?

When there is only the experience of gratification, then there is no impetus for internalization (because nothing needs to be mastered) and no laying down of healthy psychic structure.

When there is the experience of nontraumatic frustration (frustration-against-a-backdrop-of-gratification that can be worked through and mastered), then this is the occasion for the laying down of healthy psychic structure. Nontraumatic frustration is the hero in this piece.

When there is the experience of traumatic frustration (frustration that cannot be worked through and mastered), then there is no laying down of healthy structure. Traumatic frustration is the villain in this piece. We will see that traumatic frustration results in deficit and conflict and, therefore, fuels the resistance.

IN ORDER TO UNDERSTAND THE DEVELOPMENT OF PATHOLOGY, WHERE SHOULD WE START?

We will start with the need, the infantile need.

WHAT DO WE MEAN BY INFANTILE NEED?

We will address ourselves to two kinds of needs—physiological needs and psychological needs.

Drive theory is all about physiological needs: libidinal drives, aggressive drives, id needs. Such needs seek discharge; such needs (whether libidinal or aggressive) press for gratification, instinctual gratification, tension release. The object is a means to that end.

Self psychology, on the other hand, is all about psychological needs, variously described as object relational, developmental, or maturational. Such needs seek not discharge but objects; such needs press not for gratification but for recognition, empathic recognition.

The object is no longer simply a means to an end; rather, the object is the end.

WHAT ARE EXAMPLES OF SUCH NEEDS?

Think about the baby's orality: his libidinal and aggressive need to consume, to devour. Think about his anality: his aggressive need to oppose, to thwart. He wants gratification of his instincts, his drives, his impulses. Mere empathic recognition of the need affords little relief.

Think about the baby's developmental need to be held, soothed, and comforted by a warm, loving mother or father. Here he wants empathic responsiveness from the object.

DEVELOPMENT OF PATHOLOGY

WHAT HAPPENS WHEN THE CHILD'S INFANTILE NEEDS ARE TRAUMATICALLY FRUSTRATED?

We will explore the answer to this question from three different perspectives: (1) What happens to the infantile need itself? (2) What does not get internalized that should? and (3) What does get internalized that should not?

WITH TRAUMATIC FRUSTRATION, WHAT HAPPENS TO THE INFANTILE NEED?

We will look to self psychology to help us understand what happens when an infantile need has been traumatically frustrated.

According to self psychology, a traumatically frustrated developmental need gets dissociated and split off. It is as if the child gets it, on some level, that the parent is not going to be someone on whom he can count; and so, in order to protect himself against the possibility of further disappointment and heartache, he represses the need and buries his pain.

Over time, thwarted infantile needs not only persist but become intensified and reinforced.

Whether we are talking about the psychological needs of self theory or the physiological needs of drive theory, traumatic frustration of the infantile need results in its reinforcement.

WHAT HAPPENS TO TRAUMATICALLY THWARTED ANAL NEEDS?

The child of 2 has an age-appropriate anal need to oppose, to challenge. Through the provision of limits that thwart the unbridled expression of the child's anal needs, the parent functions as a drive regulator. If the limits provided are gentle but firm and if the child is able to master his frustration with, and anger toward, the authoritarian parent, then the child has the experience of nontraumatic frustration.

Over time and bit by bit, he will be able to internalize the limit-setting functions performed by the benevolently containing parent (in the form of internal ego and superego controls), which will enable him to modulate the intensity of his anal strivings.

If, on the other hand, the mother is too demanding, too punitive, too restrictive, too inconsistent in her limit setting, or too invested in struggling with the child, then it may well be too difficult for the child to master his rage at his mother for thwarting his anal need to oppose. In other words, if the child's anal needs are traumatically frustrated, then those needs become intensified over time.

WHAT HAPPENS TO TRAUMATICALLY THWARTED OEDIPAL NEEDS?

The little girl of 3, as another example, has an age-appropriate oedipal need to have exclusive possession of her father and to get her mother out of the way. The little girl's needs must ultimately be thwarted, but it is the message that accompanies such frustration that determines how the drives get tamed and how drive-regulatory structures get laid down in the ego and superego.

If the little girl's oedipal strivings are gently but firmly frustrated, that is, benevolently contained, and if she has the opportunity to process and master the frustration, then her incestuous and matricidal impulses become transformed, over time, into a capacity to feel good about herself as a female and to direct herself toward the actualization of her potential, with respect to both her personal and professional goals. In other words, her incestuous and matricidal impulses become transformed into the capacity to take initiative in the pursuit of her dreams—without the burden of guilt. If the little girl cannot master the thwarting of her oedipal strivings, then she will be destined always to be limited in life by her guilt.

WHAT HAPPENS TO TRAUMATICALLY THWARTED NARCISSISTIC NEEDS?

As a final example, the child of 4 has an age-appropriate narcissistic need to show off to his mother how good he is on his ice skates. If

DEVELOPMENT OF PATHOLOGY

the mother is able, for the most part, to gratify his need to be responded to in an admiring way, and fails him in only minor ways, then over time his exhibitionism will become tamed and modulated.

But if the mother is unable to gratify his need to be admired, then as an adult he will have an exaggerated need to be admired for how good he is, will perhaps be a show-off. His narcissism will have been reinforced. We speak of such needs in the adult as archaic narcissistic needs.

WHAT ARE NEUROTIC AND NARCISSISTIC NEEDS?

I am suggesting, then, that a traumatically frustrated libidinal or aggressive need becomes a neurotic need. If a 3-year-old girl has a libidinal need for her father, that's fine. But if, as an adult, she has a libidinal need to seduce every inappropriate and unavailable man in sight, that's a neurotic need.

By the same token, a traumatically frustrated developmental need becomes a narcissistic need. If a 4-year-old child is exhibitionistic and expects his mother to drop everything she's doing in order to watch him skate, that's age-appropriate. But if, as an adult, he still has the need for mirroring confirmation of just how grand he is, that's a narcissistic need.

In any event, an infantile need (whether libidinal/aggressive or developmental) that is traumatically frustrated becomes reinforced and more charged than ever.

WITH TRAUMATIC FRUSTRATION, WHAT DOES NOT GET INTERNALIZED THAT SHOULD?

We know that, according to self theory, if a child's developmental need is traumatically frustrated, then by definition the child does not master his disappointment in his parent, there is no transmuting internalization, there is no taking in of the good object, and there is no accretion of internal structure. According to self theory, then, traumatic frustration results in deficit (structural deficit) by default—because of what does not happen.

When we say, therefore, that structural deficit is a result of frustration improperly grieved, we mean that there is now impaired or absent regulatory capacity, whether of the drives (in drive theory) or of the self-esteem (in self theory).

In the above example of the 2-year-old, if the child's anal need to oppose, to challenge, is traumatically frustrated by a punitively limit-setting parent, then, because of what does not happen, the child develops a structural deficit—namely, an impaired capacity to regulate his aggressive drives internally. In other words, the child's destructive need to discharge his aggressive energy will not become transformed into a capacity to be healthily self-assertive and to direct his aggression into constructive channels.

In the above example of the 3-year-old, if the girl's oedipal need to have her father and triumph over her mother is traumatically frustrated by parents who make her feel that she is a bad person for having such impulses, then, because of what does not happen, the girl develops a structural deficit—namely, an impaired capacity to regulate her libidinal and aggressive drives internally. In other words, the girl's incestuous and matricidal impulses will not become transformed into a healthy capacity to feel good about herself as a female and to exercise initiative in the pursuit of her dreams, both romantic and professional.

In the above example of the 4-year-old, if the child's narcissistic need to be admired is traumatically frustrated by an empathically unresponsive parent, then, because of what does not happen, the child develops a structural deficit—namely, an impaired capacity to regulate his self-esteem internally. In other words, the child's exhibitionistic need to have his perfection confirmed by a mirroring selfobject will not become transformed into a healthy capacity to direct his own efforts toward mastery and an ability to derive pleasure from his own pursuits.

In summary, when an infantile need is traumatically frustrated, what does not get internalized is the good object, and the patient develops structural deficit.

HOW ARE NEED AND DEFICIT RELATED?

When a need is traumatically frustrated, it is reinforced and, because it is not transformed into capacity, a deficit develops. By the same

DEVELOPMENT OF PATHOLOGY

token, deficit (impaired capacity) creates need; the need is for the object to complete the self, to provide those functions the self is missing.

Both need and deficit, therefore, result from the experience of traumatic frustration and the failure to internalize a good object.

WITH TRAUMATIC FRUSTRATION, WHAT DOES GET INTERNALIZED THAT SHOULD NOT?

Self theory does not help us understand what does get internalized that should not when there is traumatic frustration. Self theory tells us simply that when there is traumatic frustration of a need, there is (1) reinforcement of that need and (2) creation of a structural deficit.

I would like to draw upon object relations theory—in particular, on W. Ronald D. Fairbairn, an object relations theorist of the British School—to supplement our understanding of what happens when there has been traumatic frustration and to help us understand how negative experiences are internally recorded and structuralized.

WHAT DOES FAIRBAIRN SAY ABOUT INTERNALIZATION AND STRUCTURALIZATION?

Fairbairn does not distinguish between traumatic and nontraumatic frustration, but he does propose a model for psychic development (1954) in which he suggests that when the child is frustrated by the parent, the child deals with such frustration by internalizing the bad parent. Unable to face the reality of the parental badness, unable to confront the reality of just how disappointing his parent really is, the child takes the burden of the parent's badness upon himself.

It is easier to sacrifice himself and his good feelings about himself than to sacrifice the relationship with his parent. By making himself bad, he is able to cling to the illusion of his parent as good.

I would like to propose that we use Fairbairn's theory to inform our understanding of what is internalized when the child's needs are traumatically frustrated. The child does not internalize the good object; instead, he internalizes the bad object—by taking the burden of the object's badness upon himself in the form of internal bad objects or pathogenic introjects.

I am suggesting, then, that we rely upon Kohut and self theory for our understanding of how good gets internalized (namely, by way of nontraumatic frustration) and that we rely upon Fairbairn and object relations theory for our understanding of how bad gets internalized (namely, by way of traumatic frustration).

Whereas self psychology provides an excellent model for the addition of new good structure and the transforming of pathological narcissism into healthy narcissism, it unfortunately does little to enhance our understanding of internal bad objects. We must look to object relations theory (the building blocks of which are these internal bad objects) in order to help us understand how bad objects are internalized and, once inside, can be modified.

IN SUMMARY, WHAT ARE THE THREE THINGS THAT HAPPEN WHEN THERE IS TRAUMATIC FRUSTRATION OF AN INFANTILE NEED?

1. What happens to the infantile need? It becomes reinforced.
2. What does not get internalized that should? A good object.
3. What does get internalized that should not? The bad object.

Kohut suggests that when the child's need is traumatically thwarted, it is reinforced and, because the good object is not internalized, structural deficit, in the form of impaired capacity, develops.

I am suggesting that we supplement such a view with the idea, drawn from Fairbairn, that what the child does internalize is the bad object or, more accurately, the interactional dynamic that exists between the child and his bad object. The negative interactional dynamic is internalized in the form of pathogenic introjects, pairs of pathogenic introjects.

It is the presence of conflict within these pairs, between the poles, that gives rise to the conflict in which object relations theorists are interested.

Traumatic frustration of infantile need, therefore, gives rise to both deficit (because of what does not happen) and conflict (because of what does happen).

DEVELOPMENT OF PATHOLOGY 55

WHAT, THEN, ARE WE SAYING HAPPENS WHEN THERE IS THE EXPERIENCE OF BAD AGAINST A BACKDROP OF GOOD?

Kohut believes that, when there is the experience of bad against a backdrop of good, the child, in an attempt to master the experience of bad, takes in the good that had been there prior to the introduction of the bad. Fairbairn, interestingly, is saying something quite different. He believes that when there is the experience of bad against a backdrop of good, the child, in an attempt to master the experience of bad, takes in the bad!

Kohut speaks to what happens when the experience of being failed can be worked through and mastered, that is, grieved. Kohut is speaking to what happens when there has been nontraumatic or optimal frustration.

I believe that Fairbairn is speaking to what happens when the experience of being failed cannot be worked through and mastered, that is, cannot be grieved; he is speaking to what happens when there has been traumatic frustration.

Although Kohut and Fairbairn would seem to be saying very different things about the child's attempts to master the experience of being failed, if we consider them to be addressing different situations, then we can use what each says to inform our understanding of internalization—namely, that properly grieved failures are the occasion for internalizing the good object and improperly grieved failures are the occasion for internalizing the bad object. Expressed somewhat differently, Kohut (and self theory) helps us understand the development of healthy structure; Fairbairn (and object relations theory) helps us understand the development of pathological structure.

WHAT IS THE RELATIONSHIP BETWEEN INTERNALIZATION AND SEPARATION FROM THE INFANTILE OBJECT?

When the child internalizes functions performed by the good parent, the child comes to need his parent less and less and is therefore gradually able to separate from him. In other words, the child is able to relinquish his attachment to the infantile object by way of internalizing the good.

On the other hand, the child internalizes the bad object in an attempt to master (or control) its badness; the child internalizes the bad object in an attempt to maintain the infantile attachment and to avoid separation. In other words, when the child internalizes aspects of the bad relationship with his parent, he does it in order not to have to separate from the infantile object.

Intense attachments to the internal bad object(s) replace the intense attachment to the external bad object.

WHAT EXACTLY IS THE NATURE OF THE ATTACHMENT TO THE INTERNAL BAD OBJECT?

It was object relations theory that recognized the importance of the patient's intense attachments to his internal bad objects. Those attachments fuel the patient's resistance and are part of what makes it so difficult for the patient to move forward in the treatment and in his life.

I would like to propose that both aggression (or hostility) and libido are involved. Aggression and hostility are directed toward the internal bad object because it is, after all, a bad object that has frustrated or disappointed.

But libido is also directed toward the object because a bad object is still much better than no object at all. If a bad object is all that the child has ever known, then it's best that he make do with that—because that's all there is. Furthermore, there is a libidinal investment in the object because, as bad as it is, there is still the hope that it may someday become a good object.

WHAT IS THE CLINICAL RELEVANCE OF THE PATIENT'S INTENSE ATTACHMENTS TO HIS INTERNAL BAD OBJECTS?

Clinically, it's extremely important to recognize that the patient's attachments to his internal bad objects have both negative and positive aspects, both aggressive and libidinal components. In other words, the negative parental introject is both hated and loved.

Think, for example, of the patient who has been involved in one relationship after the next with abusive men. We find out that her father sexually abused her when she was 5. She is aware of hating him and of feeling contempt for him, but she is not in touch with any positive feelings about him.

Before she can truly renounce him and, in the process, relinquish her pattern of involvement with abusive men, she must get back in touch with her long-repressed yearning to be close to him. She must eventually acknowledge that she had once loved him, before he exploited that love and broke her heart. Otherwise, she will be destined always to contaminate her present with the past as she compulsively plays out her unresolved childhood dramas in the here and now with the men she chooses to love. She will be destined always to choose good men and experience them as bad, or to choose good men and behave in such a fashion as to get them to become bad, or, simply, to choose bad men.

Or think of the patient who is scathingly self-critical and relentlessly self-denigrating. We find out that his father was a demanding, judgmental, perfectionistic man who never found fulfillment and pleasure in his own life and so lived vicariously through his son. The patient is deeply attached to his father.

Before the patient can give up his self-loathing, he must get back in touch with, and fully own, his rage at his father, his rage that his father never really loved him for who he was, set impossibly high goals for him, and unfairly demanded that he achieve the kind of perfection and happiness that the father was never able to find for himself in his own life.

Until the patient can acknowledge both the libidinal and the aggressive aspects of the tie to his father, he will be unable to let go of his self-hatred and his sense of himself as a failure.

HOW DOES FAIRBAIRN HELP US UNDERSTAND SUCH ATTACHMENTS?

I came to understand the importance of both the libidinal and aggressive attachments from reading Fairbairn (1943), who, as we know, writes that the child takes the burden of the parent's badness upon himself in order to master his disappointment in the parent and to preserve the relationship.

But Fairbairn goes on to say that once the child has internalized the bad parent, he splits it into two parts, the exciting object that offers the enticing promise of something good and the rejecting object that ultimately fails to come through and devastates. The so-called libidinal ego attaches itself to the exciting object; the libidinal ego longs for the enticing promise of relatedness. The antilibidinal ego attaches itself to the rejecting object; the antilibidinal ego is the repository for all the hatred and destructiveness that have accumulated as a result of frustrated longing.

These attachments (both libidinal and aggressive) are then repressed. The patient, unconscious of his compulsion to reenact the early-on situation of seduction and betrayal, is ever in search of love objects that can be made into exciting/rejecting objects, promising but never fulfilling. And the drama is recapitulated again and again, in the hope that perhaps this time it will be different, perhaps this time he will find gratification of his longing for contact.

So the process goes as follows: internalization, splitting, repression. The bad object is first internalized; it is then split into an exciting object and a rejecting object; and, finally, both objects, and the ego's attachments to them, are repressed.

The child's compulsive attachments to his internal bad objects (both the libidinal ego's attachment to the exciting object and the antilibidinal ego's attachment to the rejecting object) are therefore unconscious; but they powerfully affect subsequent relationships.

Before the patient can separate from his infantile objects, he will need to become aware of both the libidinal and aggressive components of his tie to them; rendering conscious the unconscious attachment will go a long way toward diffusing the intensity of the attachment.

But the patient may also have to reexperience, in the here and now, in relation to the therapist (a stand-in, of course, for the parent), some version of the original experience of pleasure and then pain, excitement and then devastation, seduction and then betrayal. Belatedly, he will have to grieve the reality of how initially enticing but ultimately rejecting his parent really was and of how deeply deceived he has always felt.

DEVELOPMENT OF PATHOLOGY

> ## HOW DO INTENSE ATTACHMENTS TO INTERNAL BAD OBJECTS FUEL THE PATIENT'S RESISTANCE TO RELINQUISHING THE INFANTILE OBJECT?

Fairbairn helps us understand that the patient is intensely attached (both libidinally and aggressively) to his internal bad objects and is, therefore, extremely reluctant to relinquish his ties to them.

Admittedly, Fairbairn was more interested in the exciting/rejecting object than he was in any other kind of parental object. But I think that we can usefully apply Fairbairn's ideas (about the exciting/rejecting object) to the situation, more generally, of the negative parental introject. Whatever the specific nature of the internalized bad parent, the patient longs for contact with the object even as the patient hates the object for having failed him. In other words, the patient's attachment to the negative parental introject, fueled as it is by both libido and aggression, will be powerfully conflicted and intensely ambivalent—and will only be given up reluctantly.

> ## WHAT ARE PATHOGENIC INTROJECTS?

In the sections above, we have been addressing ourselves to the nature of the patient's attachments to his internal bad objects. Fairbairn helps us appreciate that the patient is both libidinally (longingly) attached and aggressively (hatefully) attached to these objects—libidinally attached because the object excites and aggressively attached because the object rejects.

To supplement our understanding of internal bad objects, we will shift to a consideration of these internal bad objects from a somewhat different perspective; now our focus will be on the internal bad objects as introjective pairs, ever in a state of internal turmoil and conflict. We are thinking no longer about the nature of the patient's ties (libidinal and aggressive) to his internal bad objects but rather about the nature of the relationship itself between the poles of the introjective pairs—that relationship is an internalized version of the erstwhile external relationship between parent and child.

To this point, I have suggested that we think of pathogenic introjects as resulting from traumatic frustration of infantile need. I would now like to propose, more specifically, that we think of pathogenic introjects as internal presences that derive developmentally from internalizing the child's negative (traumatic) interactions with his parent. In other words, when the child takes the burden of the parent's badness upon himself, he does not simply internalize the bad parent; rather, he internalizes the negative interactional dynamic that had existed between himself and his parent. Negative interactions repeated again and again in the child's relationship with his parent but never mastered (that is, traumatic aspects of that relationship) are taken into the child's internal world and become part of his repertoire of internalized object relationships.

As an example, when criticism is a recurring interactional theme, it is internalized in the form of a criticizer introject and a criticizee introject. As another example, when intimidation is a recurring dynamic in the relationship between parent and child, it is internalized in the form of an intimidator introject and an intimidatee introject.

It is in this way that early-on negative interactions are internally recorded and structuralized.

The introjective pairs exist as charged, toxic, unassimilated foreign bodies; they are "felt presences" (Schafer 1968), neither really separate from the sense of self nor fully integrated into it. Some have suggested that they are like food in the stomach—they are in the stomach but not actually part of it.

WHAT DO WE KNOW ABOUT THE PATIENT'S ATTACHMENTS TO, AND IDENTIFICATIONS WITH, HIS INTERNAL BAD OBJECTS?

Let us look at how our understanding of the patient's attachments to, and identifications with, his internal bad objects has been enriched through the contributions first of Freud, then of Fairbairn, and finally of Otto Kernberg and W. W. Meissner.

DEVELOPMENT OF PATHOLOGY

> ## WITH RESPECT TO OUR UNDERSTANDING OF INTERNAL BAD OBJECTS, WHAT DOES FREUD HAVE TO SAY?

Freud writes of harshly punitive superego introjects that derive from internalizing the parent's harsh punitiveness. The experience of being criticized and punished by a harsh parent is internally recorded and structuralized in the form of negative superego introjects. Where once the parent railed against the child, now the superego rails against the ego. An internal relationship has replaced the erstwhile external relationship.

The internal bad parent takes up residence in the superego (which then becomes identified with the parental introject), but Freud does not address himself specifically to the nature of the child's attachment to this negative introject.

In fact, Freud was interested much more in the nature of the child's attachment to external good objects than in the nature of the child's attachment to internal bad objects. Freud's objects were the external objects from whom the child sought infantile gratification. He proposed that the libido remains tenaciously attached to external objects experienced as either gratifying or potentially gratifying; once the libido has cathected an object, it is reluctant to give it up. Freud (1926) suggested that this "adhesiveness of the libido" to its external good objects fuels the id resistance and the repetition compulsion.

Freud conceived, then, of the patient's compulsive attachments to his external good objects as deriving from adhesiveness of the libido. There was no real place in his theorizing, however, for the patient's compulsive attachments to his internal bad objects; nor did Freud address himself to the adhesiveness of the patient's aggression.

Freud was, after all, interested much more in development of the libido (the psychosexual line of development) than in development of the aggression. So, too, he was interested much more in external good objects than in internal bad objects, much more in the positive transference (which I refer to as the patient's relentless pursuit of infantile gratification in the transference) than in the negative transference (which I refer to as the patient's compulsive reenactments of his unresolved childhood dramas in the transference).

Freud did posit the existence of negative superego introjects deriving from identification of the superego with the critical parent (what we might describe as the shadow of the object falling upon the superego), but he did not address himself specifically to the nature of the patient's attachment to this internal bad parent.

WITH RESPECT TO OUR UNDERSTANDING OF INTERNAL BAD OBJECTS, WHAT DOES FAIRBAIRN HAVE TO SAY?

It is to Fairbairn that we must look in order to understand the actual nature of the patient's attachments to his internal bad objects. As we have already discussed, Fairbairn's magnificent contribution was in his appreciation of the fact that the patient's intense attachments to his internal bad objects are fueled by both libido (the longing for connection) and aggression (the reaction to frustration of that longing for connection).

Admittedly, Fairbairn was more interested in the exciting/rejecting parental object (the parent who offers the enticing promise of relatedness and then fails to deliver) than he was in the harshly punitive parental object, but, as I mentioned in an earlier section, I think we can use his idea that the child is attached both libidinally and aggressively to the internalized seductive/betraying parent to inform our understanding of the nature of the child's attachments, more generally, to the internal bad parent.

That the patient is both libidinally and aggressively invested in his internal bad objects fuels the patient's repetition compulsion and his resistance; that the patient is both libidinally and aggressively invested in his internal bad objects speaks to the difficulty the patient has relinquishing his attachment to them. Ultimately, the patient's attachments to his internal bad objects interfere with the patient's forward movement in the treatment and in his life.

Fairbairn's elaboration upon the nature of the child's ties to his internal bad objects is an important supplement, then, to Freud's depiction of the nature of the child's ties to his external good objects. And, although Freud believes that the patient is always in search of infantile gratification from his external objects, Fairbairn reminds us that the patient also has very intense aggressive and libidinal attachments to his internal bad objects.

In sum, although Freud talks about the id resistance as an adhesiveness of the libido, I think it is important to remember that there is also an adhesiveness of the aggression that makes it difficult for the patient to separate from his infantile objects and to overcome his compulsion to repeat what he would rather not.

Fairbairn is suggesting something else as well. Whereas Freud is talking about adhesiveness of the libido to good objects, Fairbairn is talking about adhesiveness of the libido to bad objects, in other words, the libidinal ego's libidinal (or positive) attachment to the bad object. The libidinal ego yearns for the exciting but ultimately rejecting object. Freud's adhesive attachments are libidinal in nature and are to external good objects; Fairbairn's intense attachments are both libidinal and aggressive in nature and are to internal bad objects.

I am suggesting, therefore, that adhesiveness of the libido to the external good object (about which Freud wrote) and attachment of the libido and the aggression to the internal bad object (about which Fairbairn wrote) are part of the resistance from the id and, as such, fuel the patient's repetition compulsion.

WHAT IS FREUD'S CONTRIBUTION TO OUR UNDERSTANDING OF THE RELATIONSHIP BETWEEN INTERNAL BAD OBJECTS?

Freud, in both *Mourning and Melancholia* (1917) and *The Ego and the Id* (1923), speaks of the relationship between the superego and the ego.

More specifically, in the first paper, Freud suggests that depression (melancholia) results from internalizing the lost love object. In the aftermath of the loss of the love object, the shadow of the lost object falls upon the ego (which means that part of the ego becomes identified with the lost object). Internalization is the person's defensive and adaptive reaction to the perceived loss of an ambivalently held, narcissistically cathected love object.

Where once the person raged against the abandoning object, now a part of the ego (what he later called the conscience or superego) sets itself apart from the rest of the ego (now identified with the abandoning object), sits in judgment upon it, and rages against it. Where once the subject railed against the object, now the superego rails against the ego. The result is depression.

In the second paper, Freud introduces the structural model of id, ego, and superego and writes more at length about the development of the superego. But this time he suggests not that the lost (oedipal) object becomes part of the ego but that the lost object becomes part of the superego. In essence, the shadow of the lost object falls upon the superego. Where once the object railed against the subject, now the superego rails against the ego.

In both instances, an internal relationship has replaced an external relationship. In the first instance, the person rages against himself where once he raged against the object. In the second instance, the person rages against himself where once the object raged against him.

In the first instance, the shadow of the object falls upon the ego. In the second instance, the shadow of the object falls upon the superego.

In the first instance, the ego identifies with the lost object; the superego attaches itself to the ego (the lost object) and rages against it as once the person attached himself to the external object and raged against it. In the second instance, the superego identifies with the "aggressing" lost object and now aggresses against the ego as once the object aggressed against him.

Freud does, then, suggest that an internal relationship between superego and ego replaces the erstwhile external relationship between parent and child. In the first instance, the abandoning parent takes up residence in the ego and the superego rails against it — as once the child raged against the parent. In the second instance, the critical parent takes up residence in the superego and the superego rails against the ego — as once the parent raged against the child.

But, except for Freud's depiction of a superego that provokes guilt and an ego that experiences it, Freud pays little attention to the existence of other pairs of pathogenic introjects. In other words, although Freud was interested in the relationship between a harshly punitive superego and a guilt-ridden ego, he appears to have had little interest in the existence of other kinds of interactional dynamics, little interest in the internal recording (as pathogenic structures) of recurring negative interactional themes between parent and child.

WHAT IS FAIRBAIRN'S CONTRIBUTION TO OUR UNDERSTANDING OF THE RELATIONSHIP BETWEEN INTERNAL BAD OBJECTS?

Although Fairbairn addressed himself to the relationship that develops between the patient and his internal bad objects, a relationship characterized by both love and hate, he did not address himself specifically to the relationship between the internal bad objects themselves. His interest was in the nature of the patient's attachment to the introjected parental object; like Freud, his specific interest was not in the internal recording of interactional dynamics between parent and child.

Fairbairn's internal bad objects are negative parental introjects; his internal bad objects correspond to the position of the parent in relation to the child. In Fairbairn's theory, there are no internal bad objects corresponding to the position of the child in relation to the parent.

WHAT DO KERNBERG AND MEISSNER HAVE TO SAY ABOUT THE RELATIONSHIP BETWEEN INTERNAL BAD OBJECTS?

Neither Freud nor Fairbairn, then, really takes into consideration the child's internalization of traumatic interactional themes between himself and his parent, negative dynamics repeated again and again in his relationship with the parent and never fully mastered. Neither, then, conceives of the patient's internal world as populated by pairs of pathogenic introjects, residues of the child's pathogenic relationship with his parent; neither conceives of the patient's internal world as structuralized by pairs of internal bad objects in a state of internal turmoil and conflict.

It is to object relations theorists like Kernberg and Meissner that we must look in order to understand that the internal bad objects themselves are in relationship.

Kernberg (1976) believes that it is the relationship itself between parent and child (whether positive or negative) that is internally recorded and structuralized as so-called relational configurations (self-object-affect complexes) consisting of three parts: an image of the self, an image of the object, and whatever affect characterizes the relationship between the two.

Meissner (1976, 1980) suggests that the relationship between parent and child (particularly aspects that are negative) are internally recorded and structuralized as pairs of introjects, so-called introjective configurations or introjective constellations with two poles: one pole represents the characteristic position of the powerful parent, and the other pole is complementary and represents the characteristic position of the vulnerable child.

In summary, although both Freud and Fairbairn speak of internal bad objects as deriving from internalization of the dysfunctional parent, it is Kernberg and Meissner (and other—more contemporary—relational theorists) who speak to internalization of the interactional dynamic between the parent and the child—and the creation of internal bad objects that represent not only the stance of the dysfunctional parent but also the stance of the dysfunctional child. And whereas Freud and Fairbairn speak to the existence of internal bad objects as representing the position of the dysfunctional parent, object relations theorists like Kernberg and Meissner speak to the existence of introjective pairs that represent both positions.

WHAT ABOUT THE VICTIMIZER AND VICTIM INTROJECTIVE PAIR?

The child who was repeatedly abused by his parent internalizes that dynamic in the form of a victimizer introject and a victim introject. I think it is useful here to think in terms of the victimizer introject as establishing itself in the superego proper (the conscience) and the victim introject as establishing itself in the ego. The interactional dynamic between the two is characterized by condemnation and moral outrage (from the side of the superego) and guilt (from the side of the ego).

Where once the child experienced himself as helpless in the face of the parent's abuse of him, now the ego experiences itself as guilty and morally reprehensible in relation to a harshly punitive superego.

An internal relationship has replaced the external relationship.

WHAT ABOUT THE SUPERIOR AND INFERIOR INTROJECTIVE PAIR?

The child who was constantly put down by a discounting parent internalizes that dynamic in the form of a superior introject and an inferior introject. It is useful to think in terms of the superior introject as taking up residence in the ego ideal and the inferior introject as taking up residence in the ego. The interactional dynamic between the two is characterized by contempt (from the side of the ego ideal) and shame (from the side of the ego).

Where once the child experienced himself as inadequate in the eyes of the demanding parent, now the ego experiences shame in relation to a perfectionistic ego ideal.

Indeed an internal relationship has replaced the external relationship.

HOW DO THESE INTROJECTIVE CONFIGURATIONS RELATE TO DEPRESSION?

I believe that angry (guilt-ridden) depressions, with which drive theorists concern themselves, speak to a discrepancy between the ego and the superego (or conscience), conflict between victim and victimizer pathogenic introjects. Similarly, I believe, as mentioned in an earlier section, that empty (shame-filled) depressions, with which self theorists concern themselves, speak to a discrepancy between the ego and the ego ideal, conflict between inferior and superior pathogenic introjects.

The patient who suffers from an angry depression is angry, full of both resentment and guilt, and experiences himself as bad, morally reprehensible. His wish is to confess his guilt and to expose his badness. The patient who suffers from an empty depression is empty, despairing, full of shame, and experiences himself as defective, inferior, and worthless. His need is to conceal his shame and to keep hidden his deep sense of himself as inadequate and a failure.

Along these same lines, it was Kohut who suggested that guilty man is to drive theory what tragic man is to self theory. Guilty man suffers from an angry depression; he feels guilt because of the presence of forbidden libidinal and aggressive impulses. Tragic man suffers from an empty depression; he feels shame because he has failed to live up to his potential.

HOW DOES A TWO-PERSON PSYCHOLOGY CONCEIVE OF CONFLICT?

We have referred to the tension within each introjective pair; the conflict that had existed (externally) between parent and child is experienced (internally) between the poles of the introjective pairs.

What is the name of such conflict?

In the literature, such conflict (within the introjective pairs) is either not named or, simply, described as structural conflict—inasmuch as it is conflict between pathogenic structures. But I think that calling it structural conflict is misleading. That term is already being used in the literature to describe something quite different from the conflict that exists within the introjective pairs.

In the classical literature, structural conflict is the term used to described conflict between id drive and ego defense. Such a perspective focuses on the intrapsychic configuration of conflict (or tension) between id and ego. When there is an imbalance among the various psychic structures (that is, when the id is particularly strong, the superego is particularly punitive, and the ego is particularly weak), then the ego— pressured from below by the id and from above by the superego—mobilizes whatever defenses it can in order to thwart the threatened breakthrough of the libidinal and aggressive drives.

The drive-defense model of classical psychoanalysis is thought to be a one-person theory of therapeutic action because it speaks to conflict within the psyche between the id and the ego.

But should we not have a way to distinguish the conflict of a two-person or interpersonal theory (the conflict within pairs of pathogenic introjects deriving from internalized external relationships) from the conflict of a one-person theory (the conflict between id and ego)?

Stephen Mitchell (1988), an object relations theorist, has suggested that the conflict within the pairs of introjects be called relational conflict, to distinguish it from the structural conflict of a one-person theory.

IS RELATIONAL CONFLICT THOUGHT TO BE CONVERGENT OR DIVERGENT?

The structural conflicts of classical psychoanalysis are convergent conflicts, conflicts of defense involving conflict between one force pressing "Yes" and another force, gathered to oppose it, countering with a "No."

With respect to the relational conflicts of object relations theory, such conflicts are divergent conflicts, conflicts of ambivalence involving a vying for supremacy of mutually exclusive forces, an either-or situation in which either one or the other will ultimately prevail.

TRAUMATIC FRUSTRATION RESULTS IN WHAT KIND OF CONFLICT?

Earlier we had said that traumatic frustration by the parent of the infantile need results in (1) reinforcement of the need; (2) deficit (because of what does not get internalized); and (3) conflict (because of what does get internalized).

The deficit that develops is, of course, structural deficit; what does not get internalized is, of course, the good object.

But what is the nature of the conflict that arises because of what does get internalized? Is it structural conflict or relational conflict? When the relationship between parent and child is traumatically frustrating, as we have just seen, the child internalizes that interactional dynamic in the form of pairs of pathogenic introjects; where once the (external) conflict was between parent and child, now the (internal) conflict is within the pairs—thereby creating relational conflict.

But, as it happens, traumatic frustration by the parent of the infantile need results also in structural conflict—although not specifically because of what does get internalized. Traumatic frustration results in a reinforcement of the id and, because of failure to internalize the good parental object, a weakened ego (and impaired capacity); as a result, the ego is forced to rely upon whatever defenses it can muster in order to keep a lid on the id—thereby creating structural conflict. Of course, the situation is more urgent when the superego, ever a thorn in the ego's side, is particularly harsh, which will be the case when the bad (traumatically frustrating) parental object is internalized and takes up residence in the superego.

And so it is that traumatic frustration results in structural deficit and both structural conflict (from the perspective of a one-person psychology) and relational conflict (from the perspective of a two-person psychology).

Expressed in somewhat different terms, traumatic frustration—the villain in this piece—results in structural deficit (with which self psychology is concerned), structural conflict (with which classical psychoanalysis is concerned), and relational conflict (with which object relations theory is concerned).

WHY DOES THE PATIENT HAVE NEGATIVE MISPERCEPTIONS OF HIMSELF AND OTHERS?

With respect to the relational conflict of object relations theory, the pathogenic introjects become part of a road map by which new experience is interpreted and given meaning. They color and distort the patient's perceptions of himself and, when projected, his perceptions of others. When both poles of an introjective configuration are kept inside, the conflict remains an internal one. But when one or the other pole is externalized, the battleground becomes an external one.

When a pathogenic introject is delivered, under the sway of the repetition compulsion, into the relationship with the therapist, the negative interactional dynamic that had characterized the earlier relationship with the parent becomes recapitulated in the (negative) transference—and the conflict is externalized.

The tip-off that projection and negative transference are involved is the fact of the patient's distorted perceptions of himself

DEVELOPMENT OF PATHOLOGY

and/or the therapist. Whenever a patient experiences either himself or his objects in an unrealistically negative light ("I am bad" or "You are bad"), then we implicate the pathogenic introjects that populate the patient's internal world and that derive from internalizing the badness that had existed in the early-on toxic relationship between the patient and his parent.

The patient's distorted perceptions speak also, of course, to ungrieved early-on losses. As we remember, had the child been able to confront the fact of the parental badness, then he would not have had to take the burden of that badness upon himself and would not now be experiencing his world (and himself) in such a distorted fashion.

SIX

Working with the Transference

HOW DOES A NEGATIVE TRANSFERENCE DEVELOP?

Whether we are thinking in terms of superior/inferior pathogenic introjects or victimizer/victim pathogenic introjects or any other introjective configuration, the conflict within the pairs is a closed system to which we have no access until it becomes externalized.

When the patient delivers his pathology into the transference, by way of projection, we have a recapitulation in the here and now of the negative interactional dynamic that had characterized the early-on traumatic failure situation between parent and child. We have, in other words, development of a negative transference.

It is important that the patient be able to deliver his pathology, in the form of his internal demons, into the transference so that we can gain access to what would otherwise have remained a closed system. We cannot effect structural change and the giving up of distortion until we have gained such access.

Because we conceive of the patient's internal world as populated by pairs of pathogenic introjects (the parental-pole and the child-pole), it stands to reason that there will be two different kinds of negative transference: the patient can activate and project onto the therapist either of the poles in the introjective pair; he will then identify with the complementary pole. In other words, the patient delivers his pathology into the treatment situation by externalizing either side of his conflict.

WHAT IS A DIRECT TRANSFERENCE?

I would suggest that we call it a direct transference when the patient re-creates with the therapist the same interactional dynamic that had characterized the earlier traumatic relationship with the parent. A direct transference unfolds when the patient projects onto the therapist the introject corresponding to the position that the powerful parent had in relation to the patient as a child; he identifies with the complementary pole and experiences himself in relation to the now powerful therapist as the vulnerable child he once was.

WHAT IS AN INVERTED TRANSFERENCE?

On the other hand, an inverted transference develops when the patient re-creates with the therapist the inverse of the dynamic that had characterized the earlier traumatic relationship with the parent. An inverted transference emerges, therefore, when the patient projects onto the therapist the introject corresponding to the vulnerable position that the patient had as a child in relation to the powerful parent; he identifies with the complementary pole and now does unto his vulnerable therapist what was once done unto him by his powerful parent.

In an inverted transference situation, the patient becomes the traumatically frustrating parent he once had and puts the therapist in the position of the traumatically frustrated child he once was; the patient repeats in the transference the early-on traumatic failure situation (this time with the roles reversed) so that the therapist can come to know, deeply, what it was really like for the patient as a child.

WORKING WITH THE TRANSFERENCE

WHAT IS AN EXAMPLE OF AN INVERTED TRANSFERENCE?

By way of illustrating an inverted transference, let us imagine a patient who has suffered terribly at the hands of a parent who was constantly putting him in no-win, double-bind situations. By doing to the therapist what was once done unto him by his double-binding parent, such a patient may be able to make the therapist feel that, no matter what the therapist does, nothing good will come of it; the therapist is made to feel the paralysis, the helpless frustration, and the impotent rage that is the story of the patient's life.

HOW ARE NEGATIVE TRANSFERENCES RESOLVED?

Let us now discuss, briefly, the process by which a negative transference is worked through. We will approach the working-through process from both a one-person perspective (wherein the interpretation is thought to be the primary therapeutic agent) and a two-person perspective (wherein the relationship between patient and therapist is thought to bring about the cure). Whether the emphasis is on the interpretation or the "real relationship," resolution of the negative transference is thought to be effected when the patient is able to let go of his distorted perceptions of both the therapist and himself in relation to the therapist.

HOW DOES A ONE-PERSON THEORY CONCEIVE OF RESOLUTION OF THE NEGATIVE TRANSFERENCE?

In a one-person theory of therapeutic action, the therapist, in order to correct the patient's distortions, offers interpretations that direct the patient's attention inward and backward, direct him to observe his internal process and the fact of his unconscious repetitions, his tendency to experience new good objects as old bad ones.

The therapist's interpretations encourage the patient to recognize that he does rather tend to make assumptions about his contemporary objects based on his experience of his infantile objects. The patient gains insight into the extent to which his perceptions of reality are contaminated by his compulsive need to experience the present in ways determined by the past.

The therapist does not specifically address the reality of the situation. He does not specifically address whether the patient's perceptions of him as bad are accurate or not. Rather, the therapist (in the form of an interpretation) simply calls the patient's attention to the fact that the patient does rather tend to make assumptions about the present based on his past.

The net result is the rendering conscious of something that had been unconscious, a strengthening of the ego, an extending of its province. Insight and increased self-awareness are achieved.

So, in a one-person theory, insight by way of interpretation is thought to be the corrective for the transference distortion.

HOW DOES A TWO-PERSON THEORY CONCEIVE OF RESOLUTION OF THE NEGATIVE TRANSFERENCE?

In a two-person theory, on the other hand, the relationship itself is thought to be the primary therapeutic agent. Accordingly, the therapist, in order to correct the transference distortions, encourages the patient to look outward in order to experience the reality of who the therapist actually is—namely, that the therapist is a new good object.

The patient must come to a point where he can recognize that there is a discrepancy between what is, in fact, real and what he had imagined was real, a discrepancy between reality on the one hand and his distortion on the other.

The patient's perception of the split between his knowledge of the therapist (informed by the present) and his experience of the therapist (informed by the past) is what eventually provides the impetus for change. It is the internal tension created through the patient's awareness (and experience) of that discrepancy that will provide the motive force for change.

So, in a two-person theory, the real relationship is thought to be the corrective for the transference distortion.

WORKING WITH THE TRANSFERENCE

In summary, I would suggest that we think of resolution of the negative transference as involving a combination of both insight (achieved by way of interpretation) and a corrective emotional experience (achieved by way of the real relationship between patient and therapist). To help us conceptualize the working-through process, therefore, we will draw upon concepts from both one-person and two-person theories of therapeutic action.

WHAT ARE THE TWO INTERNAL RECORDS OF TRAUMATIC FRUSTRATIONS?

To this point I have been suggesting that there are two internal records of traumatic frustrations sustained by the patient in his early-on relationship with his parent: (1) reinforced infantile need (and accompanying deficit) because of what does not get internalized—namely, the good parental object; and (2) internal bad objects because of what does get internalized—namely, the interactional dynamic between the patient and the bad parental object. As we earlier observed, need and deficit are both the result of a failure to internalize the good object; they are flip sides of the same coin.

The presence of infantile need gives rise to the hope that each object encountered subsequently will be the good parent the patient never had. The presence of internal bad objects gives rise to the fear that each object encountered subsequently will be the bad parent the patient did have.

HOW DOES THIS RELATE TO THE UNFOLDING OF THE TRANSFERENCE?

Under the sway of the repetition compulsion, the patient delivers both his wish for good and his fear of bad into the relationship with the therapist. The wish for good is delivered by way of displacement (displacement of need); the fear of bad is delivered by way of projection (projection of pathogenic introject).

Both situations involve a recapitulation of the past in the

present; both are instances therefore of transference, whether we are talking about displacement or projection. I suggest that we think of a positive transference as unfolding when the patient displaces his reinforced infantile needs from his parent to his therapist and that we think of a negative transference as unfolding when the patient projects his internal bad objects or pathogenic introjects onto his therapist.

In the context of the transference relationship, therefore, the patient comes both to hope for the best (through displacement of his reinforced needs) and to expect the worst (through projection of his internal bad objects). In other words, he delivers his pathology—both his wish for good and his fear of bad—into the transference, in the form of his illusions and his distortions.

WHAT IS THE RELATIONSHIP BETWEEN POSITIVE AND NEGATIVE TRANSFERENCE?

The illusions and the distortions go hand in hand because they operate on different levels. At the same time that the patient expects (through projection of his underlying pathogenic introjects) criticism, disapproval, abandonment, abuse, and so on, on another level he hopes (through displacement of his infantile needs) for gratification and clings to the illusion that the goodies will someday be forthcoming. The patient expects the worst but meanwhile continues to hope for the best.

WHAT IS THE RELATIONSHIP BETWEEN POSITIVE TRANSFERENCE AND HOPE?

The delivery, by way of displacement, of the infantile need into the relationship with the therapist creates the illusion that the therapist will be the good parent the patient never had. Such transferences are positive and are accompanied by the wish that maybe this time the patient will be gratified in ways that he was not as a child. These transferences are accompanied by hope.

If the displaced infantile needs are narcissistic, then the transference that unfolds is called a narcissistic or selfobject transference. If the displaced infantile needs are neurotic, then the transference that emerges is called a neurotic transference. But whether the transference is narcissistic or neurotic, it is accompanied by positive affect and by the hope that maybe this time the patient will be gratified in ways that he was not as a child.

WHAT IS THE RELATIONSHIP BETWEEN NEGATIVE TRANSFERENCE AND FEAR?

Very different is the situation in which the patient projects his pathogenic introjects onto the therapist and comes to fear that he will now be frustrated in the very same ways that he was once frustrated as a child.

The delivery, by way of projection, of the internal bad objects into the relationship with the therapist creates the distorted perception that the therapist will be the bad parent the patient actually had. Negative transferences are accompanied by anger, fear, hopelessness, and/or despair.

WHICH TRANSFERENCES DO WE INTERPRET?

The clinical implications of the distinction between a positive transference and a negative transference are profound. When the patient is hoping that the therapist will be the good parent he never had, we do not, for the most part, interpret such a transference. We allow it to be. Inevitably, the therapist will empathically fail the patient. It will be the disruptions of the positive transference, occasioned by these empathic failures, that will call for interpretation and working through.

On the other hand, when the patient is experiencing the therapist as the bad parent he did have (or fearing that the therapist will turn out to be the bad parent he did have), we do interpret such a transference because we want it resolved. As long as it goes uninterpreted, the patient will be in the position of reexperiencing in the here and now the same trauma experienced early on at the hands of the toxic parent. Negative transferences recapitulate the early-on traumatic failure situation and need to be worked through in order not to retraumatize the patient.

We analyze, therefore, both the negative transference and disruptions of the positive transference.

WHAT IS THE DISTINCTION BETWEEN A POSITIVE TRANSFERENCE DISRUPTED AND A NEGATIVE TRANSFERENCE?

In both situations (negative transferences and disruptions of the positive transference), the patient's affective experience will be one of dysphoria—upset, disappointment, sadness, hurt, anger, outrage. But in the instance of a negative transference, the patient's negative affect has to do with the patient's experience of the therapist as the bad parent he had feared the therapist would be. In the instance of a disrupted positive transference, the patient's negative affect has to do with the patient's experience of the therapist as having failed to be the good parent he had hoped the therapist would be—it involves the patient's disillusionment.

In the first instance, the negativity has to do with the bad that is; in the second instance, the negativity has to do with the good that is not.

In the first instance, the negativity has to do with unrealistic perception of the therapist; in the second instance, the negativity has to do with realistic perception of the therapist.

By way of example, if the patient is upset because the therapist has not given him the "magic answer" he had wanted, it may have to do with either a misinterpreting of the therapist's underlying motivations or an accurate assessment of the therapist's very real limitations. The patient may be experiencing the therapist in a distorted fashion as punitively withholding (as the parent once was) or may be experiencing the therapist realistically as less omniscient than the patient would have wished him to be.

The first instance is a situation of distortion, inaccurate perception, and negative transference; the second instance is a situation of

WORKING WITH THE TRANSFERENCE

disillusionment, accurate perception, and disrupted positive transference.

In other words, the patient may be upset because things are as he had feared they might be and/or because things are not as he had hoped they would be.

WHY IS SUCH A DISTINCTION IMPORTANT?

Often both negative transference and disrupted positive transference are involved at the same time. It is important that the therapist be able to distinguish between them because the working-through process is different for each. Whereas working through a disrupted positive transference involves, ultimately, modulating infantile need and letting go of the illusions arising from such need, working through the negative transference involves, ultimately, modifying internal bad objects and letting go of the distortions created by these pathogenic structures.

WHAT IS AN IDEALIZING TRANSFERENCE?

To highlight the distinction between a positive transference and a negative transference and the implications for treatment, let us look at an idealizing transference. Is such a transference the result of displacement or projection, displacement of the need for perfection (in this case, the need for an idealized selfobject) or projection of the superior pathogenic introject?

Let us think first about the idealizing transference that develops as a result of displacement. When there is displacement of the need for an idealized selfobject, the therapist is experienced as the embodiment of idealized perfection and then fused with in fantasy; in that way does the patient partake of the therapist's grandness— "You are perfect and I too become perfect through my fusion with you." The accompanying affect is of pleasure; the patient is being narcissistically gratified, in the sense that his experience of himself as perfect is being reinforced.

Let us compare this to the transference that develops as a result of projection. When we have the introjective pair of superior (which resides in the ego ideal) and inferior (which resides in the ego), there is tension between the two poles. As we discussed earlier, when such a pair is present, the ego tends to experience itself as a failure in the eyes of the perfectionistic ego ideal.

If the superior pole is projected onto the therapist and the conflict externalized, the patient feels shame and experiences himself as inferior in relation to the therapist. Although idealized, the therapist is seen as someone who reinforces the patient's feelings of inadequacy and defectiveness. The accompanying affect is, therefore, of anguish; and the patient is not at all narcissistically gratified.

I do not think that this second transference, which derives from projection, should be considered an idealizing transference. I think that when one speaks of an idealizing transference, one tends to mean the first situation (of displacement), although this is not always spelled out.

In the first situation, the patient feels good. Such transferences are positive and should not be interpreted—that is, not until they are disrupted, which will happen inevitably. It is important that the patient be allowed to have the experience of gratification afforded by a positive transference.

In the second situation, the patient feels bad. Such transferences are negative and are a repetition in the here and now of the early-on traumatic failure situation. They should be interpreted, because they retraumatize the patient and reinforce his bad feelings about himself.

It is important, therefore, to distinguish between these two kinds of transference. In the first situation, the narcissistic need for perfection is displaced onto the therapist. The therapeutic work that needs to be done, ultimately, is transformation of the need for perfection into a capacity to tolerate imperfection. The transformation is the result of working through a disrupted positive transference; this is what structural growth—the adding of new good—is all about.

In the second situation, the superior introject is projected onto the therapist, and the patient identifies himself with the inferior pole. The therapeutic work that needs to be done, ultimately, is detoxification of the pathogenic introjects (both poles). The detoxification is the result of working through the negative transference; this is what structural modification—the changing of old bad—is all about.

> **HOW ARE WE TO UNDERSTAND THE PROCESSES BY WHICH NEW GOOD IS ADDED AND OLD BAD IS CHANGED?**

To understand how it is that psychic structures (be they self-regulatory or drive-regulatory) are mapped out to begin with, we will be looking to self theory and what it tells us about the working through of positive transferences disrupted.

To understand how it is that existent pathological structures can be modified, we will be looking to object relations theory and what it tells us about the working through of negative transferences.

> **HOW DOES SELF PSYCHOLOGY INFORM OUR UNDERSTANDING OF STRUCTURAL GROWTH?**

Self psychology details beautifully the relationship between working through, or grieving, the loss of transference illusions and the laying down of healthy structure. From self theory, we know that optimal disillusionment is the process by which transmuting internalizations and structural growth occur.

I will be suggesting that the process of adding new good (whether self structure or drive structure) involves, ultimately, the working through of positive transferences disrupted — and self psychology informs our understanding of this process.

> **HOW DOES OBJECT RELATIONS THEORY INFORM OUR UNDERSTANDING OF STRUCTURAL CHANGE?**

Object relations theory suggests that working through transference distortions is the way underlying pathological structures (in the form of internal bad objects or pathogenic introjects) are modified.

A later chapter is devoted to the process by which pathogenic introjects are gradually detoxified and structural modification occurs. For now, let it be said that object relations theory, particularly that of Melanie Klein (1964, 1975), conceives of the (negative) transference in a dynamic sense as involving a series of cycles of projection and introjection.

The patient projects a pathogenic introject onto the therapist who, although perhaps initially accepting of the projection, ultimately challenges it (when it turns out that the therapist is not, in fact, as bad as the patient had feared he would be). The patient now reintrojects a slightly modified introject—an amalgam, part contributed by the patient (the original projection) and part contributed by the therapist (who lends some of his otherness to the interaction, so that what the patient reinternalizes will contain aspects of something new and good as well as something old and bad).

Whereas the patient may have projected out something that was 100 percent bad, what he introjects (because of the therapist's contribution) may be only 99 percent bad. The patient then projects out 99 percent bad; because of the therapist's challenging of it, what the patient reintrojects may now be only 98 percent. And so forth.

WHAT ARE SERIAL DILUTIONS?

I refer to this process of gradual detoxification of pathogenic structures as "serial dilution." Eventually, the pathogenic structures (the pathogenic introjects or internal bad objects) become more reality-based; as this happens, the negative transference begins to resolve—where once the patient needed to see the therapist as bad, now the patient develops the capacity to experience the therapist more realistically. In other words, by way of ongoing and repetitive serial dilutions, the underlying pathogenic structures are reworked and assimilated as healthy capacity.

I suggest, therefore, that the process of changing old bad involves, ultimately, the working through of negative transferences—and object relations theory informs our understanding of this process.

WHEN, AND TO WHAT EXTENT, IS THE THERAPIST (IN HIS CAPACITY AS A TRANSFERENCE OBJECT) EXPERIENCED AS A NEW GOOD OBJECT OR AS AN OLD BAD ONE?

Many have suggested that an important part of the healing that takes place in therapy has to do with the fact that the therapeutic setting is a symbolic recreation of the early-on relationship between mother and child.

But what do they really mean? Do they mean the creation of a new, good relationship unlike anything the patient has ever before experienced? Or do they mean the recreation of the old, bad relationship that the patient actually did experience with his mother?

In fact, sometimes they mean the creation of something new and good (as with the deficiency-compensation model espoused by such theorists as Michael Balint [1968], Harry Guntrip [1973], and Kohut [1971, 1977, Kohut and Wolf, 1978]) and sometimes they mean the re-creation of something old and bad (as with the relational-conflict model espoused by such theorists as Merton Gill [1982, 1983], Edgar Levenson [1983], Hans Loewald [1960], Meissner [1976, 1980], Mitchell [1988], Heinrich Racker [1968], and Joseph Sandler [1987]).

WHAT IS THE DEFICIENCY-COMPENSATION MODEL OF THERAPEUTIC ACTION?

The deficiency-compensation model conceives of the therapeutic setting as creating symbolically an ideal mother-child relationship. The therapist provides a holding environment that fosters growth, a symbolic creation of an ideal mother-child relationship very different from the pathogenic mother–child relationship the patient actually had.

A deficiency-compensation model believes in the importance of providing some degree of gratification of the patient's needs. A number of those who embrace the deficiency-compensation model of therapeutic action believe that it is the experience of gratification itself that is compensatory and ultimately healing.

Others, however, believe that it is the experience of frustration against a backdrop of gratification that promotes structural growth. Such theorists claim that if there is no thwarting of desire (no frustration), then there is nothing that needs to be mastered and, therefore, no impetus for internalization. These theorists (mostly self psychologists) believe that it is the experience of being failed and of grieving such failure that is ultimately reparative.

As patients become for themselves the good parent they never had, their need to have their objects be other than who they are becomes transformed into a capacity to accept them as they are, imperfect to be sure but nonetheless plenty good enough. Their transferential need for the good parent they never had becomes transformed into a mature capacity to know and accept their objects as they are, uncontaminated by the need for them to be otherwise.

WHAT IS THE RELATIONAL-CONFLICT MODEL OF THERAPEUTIC ACTION?

The relational-conflict model, on the other hand, conceives of the therapeutic setting as re-creating the actual bad relationship that this particular patient had with his toxic mother. Now the therapeutic setting offers the patient an opportunity to re-create in the here and now the early-on environmental failure situation, an opportunity to relive, to reexperience, indeed, to repeat, within the patient-therapist relationship, the original trauma.

But this time, because the therapist is not, in fact, as bad as the parent had been, there can be a different outcome. This time, because the therapist has capacity where the parent did not, it will be different. It will be repetition of the original trauma but with a much healthier resolution—the repetition leading to modification of the patient's internal world and integration on a higher level.

In other words, when the patient has had the experience of "not enough good" early on, then the patient must have the opportunity to experience "new good" in the relationship with the therapist. But when the patient has had the experience of "too much bad" early on, then it is not enough that the patient have the opportunity to experience "new good." Rather, the patient must have the opportunity to rework the internalized badness by experiencing first "old bad" in the relationship with the therapist and then "bad made good."

WHY DOES THE PATIENT NEED BOTH A NEW GOOD OBJECT AND AN OLD BAD ONE?

Jay Greenberg (1986) has written: "If the analyst is not seen as a new object, the analysis never begins; if not as an old one, the analysis never ends" (p. 98) — which captures exquisitely the delicate balance between the therapist's provision of something new and good (so that there can be a starting over or a new beginning) and the therapist's provision of something old and bad (so that there is opportunity for belated mastery, a reworking of internal pathogenic structures).

Greenberg's quotation also speaks to the dynamic tension between positive transference and negative transference, the dynamic tension between the patient's experience of the therapist as a new good object and his experience of the therapist as an old bad one.

I am suggesting, in essence, that patients have both a healthy need for the therapist to be the good parent they never had (which fuels the positive transference) and a healthy need for the therapist to be the bad parent they did have (which fuels the negative transference). In other words, patients have a transferential need to get the therapist to be a new good object (so that they can have now what they never had as a child) and a transferential need to get the therapist to be the old bad object (so that they can rework the original trauma and transform it).

II

Clinical Interventions

SEVEN

Listening to the Patient

DOES THE PATIENT WANT TO BE UNDERSTOOD OR TO UNDERSTAND?

There are times when all the patient wants is empathic recognition. There are other times, however, when the patient is interested in acquiring insight. It is for the therapist, moment by moment, to ascertain whether the patient wants to be understood or wants to understand. The therapist must be ever attuned to, and respectful of, the tension, the delicate balance within the patient between these two needs.

CAN YOU SAY MORE ABOUT WHEN THE PATIENT WANTS TO BE UNDERSTOOD?

Sometimes the patient is experiencing something very deeply and wants, simply, to be understood, to have what he's feeling appreciated and validated.

He may, for example, be totally immersed in a compulsive reenactment with his therapist of an unresolved childhood drama and have no interest whatsoever in understanding the part he plays in what is happening. At such times it behooves the therapist not to badger the patient with premature interpretations about the possible meaning of the patient's behavior nor to encourage the patient to reflect upon his participation in the dramatic reenactment; rather, the therapist must appreciate that the patient wants empathic recognition of the upset, anger, fear, or pain that he is feeling.

The therapist must be able to convey to the patient that he is listening and that he does understand — perhaps how frantic the patient feels, perhaps how confused, perhaps how victimized, perhaps how helpless, perhaps how desperate he is. All these feelings may well have arisen in the context of what the patient is himself doing, but the patient does not yet know this, nor does he yet care to know.

Although the therapist might wish that the patient were interested in understanding the role he plays in the unfolding of his life's dramas, the patient simply may not, at this point, be all that interested. In such situations, insight and understanding are more a priority for the therapist than they are for the patient. They speak to the therapist's agenda, not the patient's. The therapist must be respectful of the patient's need not to know; if he listens well, he will appreciate that the patient, for whatever the reason, is needing in the moment not to know.

WHAT DID BALINT AND WINNICOTT HAVE TO SAY ABOUT THE THERAPIST'S STANCE IN RELATION TO THE PATIENT?

Balint (1968) encouraged therapists to assume an "unobtrusive" stance, so that the patient would be able "to discover his way to the

LISTENING TO THE PATIENT

world of objects—and not be shown the 'right' way by some profound or correct interpretation" (p. 180). And D. W. Winnicott (1958) observed that, as he had become more experienced, he had learned to be more patient and to wait, resisting his temptation to ply the patient with clever interpretations. He had come to understand, he said, that his interpretations often did more to show the patient the limits of what he knew than anything else.

CAN YOU SAY MORE ABOUT WHEN THE PATIENT WANTS TO UNDERSTAND?

Sometimes, however, the patient does become curious about his internal process and is then interested not only in being understood but also in understanding. He may find himself wanting to understand the part he plays in his life's dramas and may, at such times, be very receptive to the therapist's interventions.

HOW DOES THE THERAPIST DECIDE WHETHER THE PATIENT WANTS TO BE UNDERSTOOD OR TO UNDERSTAND?

Basically, the therapist uses his intuition to determine where the patient is in the moment. Ever mindful of the conflict within the patient between his desire to be understood and his desire to understand, the therapist listens empathically to the patient in order to assess the patient's readiness for interventions that will highlight the patient's sense of himself as agent and not victim. The therapist uses his intuition to find those moments when there are such windows of opportunity, those moments when the patient has the capacity for insight.

There are times, then, when we find ourselves answering some of the patient's questions; but there are other times when we sense that there is a window of opportunity to encourage the patient to become curious about the internal workings of his mind—Where does his question come from? What is he really wanting to know? And why now?

There are times when we provide reassurance to the patient who clamors for it; but there are other times when we ask that the patient look at his internal process — Why the need to get reinforcement from the outside? Why such insistence? And what does it say about his experience of himself and his objects?

In other words, there will be times when we choose, simply, to gratify the patient's need; but there will be other times when we wonder, with the patient, about why he feels the need.

HOW DOES THE THERAPIST POSITION HIMSELF IN RELATION TO THE PATIENT?

It is important, therefore, that the therapist be ever attuned, on a moment-by-moment basis, to whether the patient is interested in having his experience understood or is interested in observing his experience and understanding it. And so the therapist must decide from moment to moment whether:

1. to be with the patient where he is (when the therapist senses that what the patient most wants is to be understood) or
2. to direct the patient's attention to elsewhere (when the therapist senses that the patient wants to understand).

HOW DOES THE THERAPIST'S STANCE IN RELATION TO THE PATIENT AFFECT THE LEVEL OF THE PATIENT'S ANXIETY?

When the therapist is with the patient where he is, he eases the patient's anxiety. When the therapist directs the patient's attention elsewhere, he raises the patient's anxiety. The therapist can therefore titrate the level of the patient's anxiety by supporting the patient or challenging him, or by doing first one and then the other.

HOW DOES THE THERAPIST ENGAGE THE PATIENT'S EXPERIENCING EGO AND HIS OBSERVING EGO?

When the therapist wants to convey to the patient that he is with the patient, he addresses his interventions to the patient's experiencing

LISTENING TO THE PATIENT

ego. When the therapist decides to direct the patient's attention elsewhere, his interventions are addressed to the patient's observing ego.

For the most effective psychodynamic work to occur, the therapist needs to be able to connect with both the patient's experiencing ego and his observing ego, both the patient's heart and his head. If only his experiencing ego is engaged in the therapeutic process, then the patient will have difficulty stepping back from his experience in the moment in order to reflect upon his internal process. If only his observing ego is engaged, then the patient may be able to achieve intellectual insight but unable to translate it into emotional insight and actual change.

WHAT DOES WORKING THROUGH THE RESISTANCE MEAN?

I think that the most effective game plan is one in which the therapist alternates between being with the patient where he is and directing the patient's attention elsewhere, between engaging the patient's experiencing ego and engaging the patient's observing ego, between encouraging the patient's elaboration of his subjective reality — his characteristic (defensive) posture in the world — and reminding the patient about what he (the patient) really does know to be objective reality.

Back and forth, back and forth, over and over again. Systematically, repeatedly, again and again. The therapist weaves a web, in and out, back and forth, first what the patient experiences and then what the patient knows, and then once again back to what the patient experiences, and so forth. This is what is meant by working through the resistance. It is a process that requires of the therapist that he be able to demonstrate to the patient the same thing again and again, at different times, and in different contexts. Recurring patterns, themes, repetitions. Here too. Here now. Here also.

DOES THE THERAPIST ADDRESS HIMSELF TO THE PRESENT, THE TRANSFERENCE, OR THE PAST?

Not only must the therapist decide, from moment to moment, whether to be with the patient where he is or to direct his attention elsewhere, but also the therapist must decide, moment by moment, whether to address his interventions to the patient's present, the transference, or the past.

Karl Menninger (1958) has suggested that when the patient is talking about what's going on with respect to current objects, the therapist should be with the patient in that and then, when the moment is right, direct the patient's attention to the transference. When the patient is talking about what's going on in the transference, the therapist should be with the patient in that and then, when the time is opportune, direct the patient's attention to the past, to his infantile objects. After the patient has understood something further about his past and its impact on him in the here and now, the patient may then, of his own accord, revert to talking about what's going on for him in his present reality, but now with a deeper level of awareness and understanding of how the present is informed by the past. This progression (from the present to the transference to the past and then back to the present again) is referred to as Menninger's triangle of insight.

WHY IS IT IMPORTANT THAT THE THERAPIST BE ABLE TO DECENTER?

As the therapist sits with the patient, he tries as best he can to decenter from his own experience of the world and, instead, to enter into the patient's experience of it — so that he can come to know the world as the patient knows it, uncontaminated by his (the therapist's) own perspective.

WHAT IS THE DISTINCTION BETWEEN EASY EMPATHY AND DIFFICULT EMPATHY?

It is relatively easy for someone to empathize with people like himself, much harder to empathize with people unlike himself. When the patient experiences the world as the therapist experiences it and reacts as the therapist would react, it is not too difficult for the therapist to enter into the patient's experience and to be with him in that. But when the patient is really different from the therapist, then it is a lot more difficult for the therapist to enter into the patient's experience and to understand, deeply, why the patient feels and behaves as he does.

For example, it is not too hard to be empathic with a patient who is upset because her boyfriend physically abuses her. She shows us the bruises where he has hit her and she tells us that she is frightened and angry, and we have no trouble whatsoever joining with her in her sense of outraged betrayal.

But it is much more difficult to be empathic when she now tells us that, even though he repeatedly abuses her, she cannot leave him. This latter situation requires of us that we relinquish our investment in thinking that things should be a certain way. It requires of us that we be willing to put ourselves in her place so that we can come to understand why she feels she cannot leave this man who hurts her so.

Perhaps we come to understand that, even though there are times when he makes her feel awful, there are other times when he makes her feel loved in a way that she has never before felt loved. Perhaps we come to appreciate that when he is loving her he makes her feel very special, and she is deeply grateful to him for that. Perhaps we come to see her fear that, were she to leave him, she would never find another man.

Or perhaps being in the relationship with this man enables her to cling to her hope that maybe someday, if she tries hard enough, she may yet be able to get him (a stand-in for her father) to love her as she so desperately wants to be loved. She does not like the abuse but is willing to put up with it, if it means being able to hold on to her hope that someday she may be able to get the love she has wanted for so long.

The truly empathic therapist will be able to enter deeply into the patient's internal experience and to appreciate, in a profoundly respectful way, how it is that being in the abusive relationship serves the patient—in other words, what her investment is in staying.

WHAT DOES IT MEAN TO BE TRULY EMPATHIC?

The truly empathic therapist must be ever aware of where the patient is in the moment, whether it is something the therapist can easily understand or something the therapist can understand only with great difficulty. But whether that task is easy or hard, the therapist must be able to come to the point where he can deeply appreciate why the patient needs the defenses that he has, why the patient protects himself in the ways that he does, why the patient refuses to make changes in his life, why the patient holds on to the past, and why the patient cannot let himself move forward in his life.

HOW MUCH ARE WE WITH THE PATIENT WHERE HE IS AND HOW MUCH DO WE DIRECT HIS ATTENTION ELSEWHERE?

For the most part, we strive to be with the patient where he is, validating, supporting, and reinforcing. Only when we sense that we have a window of opportunity to direct the patient's attention elsewhere do we do so. Only when we feel that the patient will be able to tolerate the temporary disconnection occasioned by our stepping away from him do we direct the patient's attention to where we would want him to be.

WHAT IS THE TECHNICAL TASK FOR THE THERAPIST?

The technical task for the therapist is to find those moments when the patient will be able to tolerate our momentary abandonment of him. The technical task for the therapist is to find those moments when we can mobilize the patient's observing ego, those moments — those windows of opportunity — when we can direct the patient's attention somewhere else.

When the patient is feeling his pain deeply, he is not usually interested in insight; what he wants is recognition, empathic recognition of his pain. Usually intense affect can be interpreted only when it has become defused a bit and the patient has achieved a certain distance from it.

So the therapist may initially need to be with the patient where he is, in his pain; and then the therapist may be able to direct the patient's attention elsewhere, so that the patient can come to understand what his pain is all about: "It hurts terribly to be so 'not seen' by Jane. I wonder if the being not seen awakens some of the old pain about how not seen you felt by your mother."

WHAT ABOUT THE RECURRING PATTERNS AND THEMES?

The patient's attention must eventually be drawn to the fact that there are recurring themes, patterns, and repetitions in his life, and that he, the patient, is the common denominator. As Menninger (1958) notes, such patterns, like the footprint of a bear that lost several of its toes in a trap long ago, stamp themselves with every step of the patient's life journey.

HOW DO WE HIGHLIGHT THE PATIENT AS AGENT?

The patient's attention is also drawn to his own activity, that it is he himself who has been bringing about what, up until then, he had thought he was experiencing passively: "The experience, then, is of being not seen by Jane, and that hurts terribly—though we are also beginning to see a pattern here, that you seem to choose narcissistic women who, like your mother, don't really listen and don't ever really get to know you."

Ultimately it is the fact of the repetition, the fact that it happens again and again, which the patient now sees, that goes a long way toward persuading the patient that in the future things no longer need to be the way they had always been in the past.

The next chapter explores, more specifically, the kinds of interventions the therapist can offer the patient who is struggling with internal conflict.

EIGHT

Responding to the Patient

WHAT ARE SOME FAIRLY TYPICAL SITUATIONS OF CONFLICT?

To demonstrate the ways in which the concepts of conflict and resistance can be applied to the clinical situation, let us think about the following three situations:

1. Clearly the patient is angry, but he denies that he is.
2. The patient knows that his therapist does not have magic, but he wishes his therapist did.
3. The patient knows that he may be limiting the benefit he can derive from his treatment by coming every other week, but he is unwilling to commit to weekly sessions.

On the one hand, there are certain realities that it would behoove the patient to acknowledge—namely, that he is angry, that his therapist does not have magic, and that he is limiting the effectiveness of his treatment by refusing to commit to more frequent sessions. On the other hand, acknowledgment of these realities makes the patient anxious and so he mobilizes any of a number of defenses to protect himself from the truth.

The therapist, in each of the above situations, has three options: (1) he can confront the patient's defense, (2) he can support it, or (3) he can do first one and then the other. From moment to moment, the therapist must decide whether he thinks it will be more useful to the patient to have his defense confronted, to have it supported, or to have the fact of his internal conflict highlighted.

HOW DO WE CHALLENGE THE PATIENT'S DEFENSE?

The therapist's first option is to come down on the side of the force that says "Yes," which supports the patient's health but makes him more anxious and, therefore, more defensive or resistant. We might therefore say:

1. "You know that some people might feel angry in such a situation."
2. "You know that I do not have magic."
3. "You know that you may be limiting the benefit you can derive from your treatment by coming every other week."

Here, in order to make the patient more aware of an anxiety-provoking reality that he both does and doesn't know, we are rather boldly naming that reality. Actually, we are naming something that the patient really does know (on some level) but against which he defends himself.

HOW DO WE SUPPORT THE PATIENT'S DEFENSE?

The second option is to come down on the side of the force that says "No," that is, go with the defense, go with the resistance, which eases

RESPONDING TO THE PATIENT

the patient's anxiety by validating his internal experience. We might then say something like:

1. "Right now you are not aware of feeling particularly angry, and, in fact, pride yourself on your ability to stay in control."
2. "You would wish that I had magic because you are so tired of having to do everything on your own."
3. "You find yourself feeling reluctant to commit to weekly sessions because you are not yet convinced that the therapy will really be able to help you."

In each of these situations, we are choosing, for the moment, to go with the resistance by naming the defense, in an experience-near, nonjudgmental, nonshaming fashion. To name the defense, we must enter so completely into the patient's internal experience that we are able to resonate with where the patient is and what really matters to him. We can then articulate, in a deeply respectful way, something about his (defensive) posture—that he takes great pride in his ability to stay in control, that he has grown weary of having to do everything on his own, or that he despairs of ever being helped by way of therapy.

WHAT HAPPENS IF WE FIRST CHALLENGE AND THEN SUPPORT THE PATIENT'S DEFENSE?

The third option is to do both—first speak to the anxiety-provoking force within the patient against which he is defending himself and then, just as he is becoming anxious, come down on the side of his resistance (in order to relieve his anxiety). And so we would say:

1. "You know that some people might feel angry in such a situation, but right now you are not aware of feeling particularly angry, and, in fact, pride yourself on your ability to stay in control."
2. "You know that I do not have magic, but you would wish that I did because you are so tired of having to do everything on your own."

3. "You know that you may be limiting the benefit you can derive from your treatment by coming every other week, but you find yourself feeling reluctant to commit to weekly sessions because you are not yet convinced that the therapy will really be able to help you."

I refer to such statements as "conflict statements." Each such statement first names a reality against which the patient defends himself and then names the thing that does the defending.

In each statement, the conflict between the patient's knowledge of reality and his experience of it is articulated. The conflict statement says, in essence, "Even though your knowledge is that . . . , nonetheless your experience is that . . ." or "Even though you know that . . . , nonetheless you feel that . . ."

WHAT, MORE SPECIFICALLY, DOES A CONFLICT STATEMENT DO?

In a conflict statement, first the therapist names the force that says "Yes," the positive force against which the patient defends himself because it creates anxiety. In the first situation above, the anxiety-provoking "Yes" force is an uncomfortable affect (anger); in the second, the anxiety-provoking "Yes" force is the recognition of a disillusioning reality—namely, that the transference object is not as good (magical) as the patient would have wanted him to be; and in the third, the anxiety-provoking "Yes" force is the acknowledgment of a sobering reality—namely, that the effectiveness of the patient's treatment may well be compromised by the patient's unwillingness to commit himself to it on a more frequent basis.

Then the therapist names the force that says "No," the negative force, the defense, the resistance. In the first situation, the patient's defense is his need to deny his anger (because feeling angry is not compatible with his sense of himself as someone who is able, for the most part, to stay in control). In the second, the patient's defense is his need to believe in magical solutions (because he is so tired of having to do everything on his own). In the third, the patient's defense is his need to hold himself back from making a commitment to weekly sessions (because of his despair about his potential to get better). The therapist names the patient's defense in a way that highlights the fact of it, without implying that there is something wrong with it.

In other words, in a conflict statement, first the therapist confronts the defense by highlighting the presence of the thing against which the patient defends himself, and then the therapist supports the defense by coming down on the side of the thing doing the defending. In the first half of the conflict statement, the thing that makes the patient anxious is named; in the second half, the thing doing the defending is named.

WHAT ARE EXAMPLES OF STATEMENTS THAT SIMPLY SUPPORT OR REINFORCE THE PATIENT'S RESISTANCE?

When our aim is to go with the resistance, we may be able to frame our interventions in such a fashion that the patient will not only feel understood but also be able to gain further understanding.

"You do not want to be in the position of needing me, or anybody."
"You are determined not to let anyone matter that much."
"You're not sure you have all that much to say about the termination."
"It's important to you that you be always in control."
"It hurts too much to think about how disappointed you are."
"It's important to you that you not let little things get to you."
"You are not sure that you have much faith in this process."
"You are not yet convinced that I can be trusted."
"You want desperately to find here the kind of understanding you were never able to find elsewhere in the past."
"You feel entitled to be compensated now for what you suffered as a child."
"You are not sure you can continue unless you can have a guarantee that this will work."

"You are wishing that I could tell you what to do."

"You are convinced that you have already done everything you can do."

"It is important to you that you be able to take care of others."

"You find yourself looking to others for the answers."

When we go with the patient's resistance, we do not challenge it. We are not interpreting the patient's stance as a defense against something else; we are simply naming it, highlighting it, defining it. It is the patient's way of constructing his world; it is the patient's way of being in relationship; it is the patient's way of being himself; it is what really matters to the patient. Ever respectful of where the patient is in the moment, we deeply appreciate that the patient has come to be as he is (and to have the defenses that he does) for good reason.

If we do not challenge the patient and his need for defense, then he may, of his own accord, begin to elaborate upon how he has come to protect himself in the ways that he does.

HOW DOES NAMING THE PATIENT'S DEFENSE RELATE TO DEFINING THE PATIENT'S CHARACTERISTIC STANCE IN THE WORLD?

When we name the patient's defense, we are really highlighting and defining the patient's basic stance in life, his characteristic (defensive) posture in the world. With our help, the patient is being encouraged to define ever more clearly the realities that he has constructed on the basis of his past experiences.

Even though they are defensive, these realities are the ways the patient tends to perceive himself and his objects; they speak to his ways of being in the world. When the therapist names the defense, the therapist is encouraging the patient to articulate some of the basic assumptions he has about himself and his objects, some of his underlying "mythological preconceptions" (Angyal 1965), in an effort to get the patient to be aware of how he structures his experience.

The patient must recognize that he perceives the world through the lenses of his need for things to be other than how they are. He must understand that he has constructed a world view that involves distortion, illusion, and entitlement, and that these misperceptions determine the ways in which he structures his experience of reality.

HOW DO WE ATTEMPT TO EMPOWER THE PATIENT?

When we name the patient's defense, we do what we can to use words that emphasize the element of choice in what the patient is feeling/doing; we want the patient, over time, to recognize and to own the power he has to decide how he makes meaning of his world.

When we suggest, for example, that the patient is determined not to cry or that he does not want to be in the position of needing anybody, we are attempting to name the power he has to make certain choices.

Think about the difference between "You do not have all that much to say about the termination" and "You are not sure that you have all that much you would want to say about the termination." Whereas the first intervention suggests that there may be something lacking in the patient (because he does not have much to say about the termination), the second intervention lends the patient a little more dignity by highlighting the element of choice in the patient's behavior.

Think about the difference between "You are not sure that you deserve good things because you are filled with such self-hatred" and "You are not sure that you deserve good things because you are filled with such hatred for yourself" or "You are not sure that you deserve good things because you hate yourself so much." Whereas the first intervention suggests that the patient is a victim of self-hatred, a static situation over which he has little control, the second and third interventions highlight the patient as agent, as someone who (actively) hates.

More generally, whenever we name the patient's defense, we want to make him ever more conscious of the volitional component in his experience of himself and his objects; in essence, we want him to move closer to owning the ways in which he (defensively) constructs himself and his world.

WHAT IS AN EXAMPLE OF SUPPORTING THE PATIENT'S DEFENSE?

Let us think about the following scenario. The patient comes to the session 5 minutes late and insists, with some vehemence, that his lateness had nothing to do with ambivalent feelings about being there and that he had very much wanted to come.

The therapist knows that the previous session had been very hard for the patient and that, despite the patient's protests to the contrary, the patient must on some level have feelings about that. The therapist could choose to explore some of those feelings. The patient, in response to the therapist's attempts to ferret out his underlying feelings, might perhaps be forthcoming about such feelings, but more probably the therapist's probing would make the patient dig in his heels, would make him even more defensive. After all, the patient had already insisted, with fairly intense affect, that his lateness had nothing to do with mixed feelings about being there.

Let us imagine that the therapist decides instead to take the patient at his word and not to insist that the patient admit to having negative feelings about the previous session. The therapist recognizes that the locus of the patient's affect in the moment is his distress, his concern that he will not be believed—thus his vehement insistence that it had been important to him to be there. And so the therapist says, "It's important to you that I understand just how much you wanted to be here today, and on time." Here the therapist is going with the resistance, by resonating, in a respectful way, with the patient's need to have the therapist believe that he had wanted very much to come. The patient will feel relieved, because the therapist has appreciated how important it was to him that he be taken at his word.

The therapist must learn to be patient; he must not need the patient to be ever busy acknowledging how he is really feeling. There will be time enough to explore the patient's underlying feelings when and as the patient becomes less anxious, less defensive.

> **HOW CAN THE THERAPIST BOTH CONVEY HIS RESPECT FOR THE PATIENT'S NEED AND HIGHLIGHT ITS DEFENSIVE ASPECT?**

Whenever we use the construction "It's important to you that _____ ," we are attempting to convey to the patient our respect for the patient's need, albeit a defensive one. But, by highlighting how important it is to the patient that his need be acknowledged, we are subtly suggesting the defensive nature of the patient's need. Without actually telling the patient that we think his need is suspect, we are nonetheless highlighting something that we want the patient eventually to notice, even as we are appreciating that, in the moment, the patient needs us to be with him.

In the above example, in response both to the patient's lateness and to his insistence that the lateness had nothing to do with anything, the therapist appreciates the patient's need to have the therapist take him, and his investment in their work together, seriously. When the therapist says to the patient, "It's important to you that _____ ," he is being profoundly respectful of the patient's need to be taken at his word.

At the same time, by highlighting the fact of its importance, the therapist is also gently suggesting that the patient's insistence that he be taken at his word is of note (and may, at some point, bear further exploration).

> **HOW, THEN, DOES THE THERAPIST CONVEY TO THE PATIENT THAT HE HAS BEEN HEARD?**

If the patient is telling us in many ways that he is feeling desperate, even suicidal, then it may well be that he is afraid he will not be heard, afraid his desperation will not be taken seriously. If the therapist says something like "It's important to you that I understand just how desperate you're feeling," then the therapist is clearly picking up on how important it is to the patient that he be able to communicate to the therapist how desperate he feels — which will ease the patient's anxiety and his fear of not being heard.

WHAT IS ANOTHER EXAMPLE OF SUPPORTING THE PATIENT'S DEFENSE?

Therapist: I wanted to let you know that I'll be away for four weeks in August.
Female patient: Oh, I'm glad you'll have a chance to get away this summer.

If the therapist were to try to interpret the id material, namely, to try to make the patient aware of her underlying feelings, he might then say something like "I think you may also be angry and upset that I'll be away for so long," to which the patient might respond with "You could be right, but I'm not aware of feeling that way."

The therapist may well be right, but if the patient opposes, as she is likely to do when such an interpretation is offered, then we've gotten nowhere and have instead created the potential for a struggle. Patients need to defend themselves now against acknowledging id material, both to themselves and to us, for the very same reason that they needed to defend themselves in the first place—namely, that acknowledgment of the underlying id content arouses too much anxiety. And so it is that the patient says defensively, "You could be right, but I'm not aware of feeling that way."

An id psychology wishes to bypass interference run by the ego in order to get to the id content. This is what Freud was all about initially (with his interest in hypnosis and the cathartic method); and it is what we, in our impatience, may sometimes unwittingly and mistakenly do with our patients. An ego psychology (in which Freud later became interested, in large part because of his introduction of the structural theory of the mind) recognizes the importance of understanding (and analyzing) the ego defense before access can be gained to the underlying id content.

In other words, if the patient says he has a secret but can't tell us, we are really more interested in why the need for the secret than in the secret itself—because the patient's investment in having a secret may be far more telling than the actual content of the secret.

So let us imagine that, in response to this patient's "Oh, I'm glad you'll have a chance to get away this summer," the therapist says, "And it's important to you that it not bother you—my being away this summer." Such a statement is attempting to highlight, in a gentle manner, the patient's ego defense, her need not to let certain kinds of things get to her. The session might then have continued along these lines:

Patient: That's right. I have always managed well on my own.

Therapist: Much of your life you have had to fend for yourself, and you have always prided yourself on how well you've done at that, on how independent you've been.

Patient: (with affect) Yes, when I was a little girl, when my parents went out they always had me look after my little brother. Nobody helped me. It was all my responsibility.

Therapist: When you were asked to be the caretaker, you did it well and you did it without complaining. Even if it did get a little lonely sometimes, you knew you could do it if you had to. (softly) So you know you can count on yourself to be able to manage just fine when I'm away in August.

Patient: (very sad, with tears) Yes.

This example provides a powerful illustration of how effective it can be when the therapist simply goes with the resistance by coming down on the side of the defense. When the therapist says, "And it's important to you that it not bother you—my being away this summer," he is letting the patient know that he understands, that he knows how important it is to the patient that she not let herself feel bad about her therapist's upcoming vacation.

The patient is then able to go on, with some affect, to elaborate upon her need for the defense—it had served her well, in her family, to be self-reliant. In time, she even came to pride herself on her ability to handle things on her own.

When the therapist says, "Even if it did get a little lonely sometimes, you knew you could do it if you had to," he is using a conflict statement (something to which I refer, more specifically, as a defense-against-affect conflict statement), first gently suggesting he knows that as a child she must have felt lonely sometimes and then respectfully acknowledging the pride she must have felt at being able to do it all on her own.

By juxtaposing the thing against which the patient defends herself because it provokes anxiety and the thing doing the defending, the therapist is able to bring more closely together the two sides of the conflict with which the patient is struggling — her sadness about being on her own and the pride she takes in being self-sufficient. But, in the face of the therapist's gentle naming of the loneliness he knows she must have felt as a child, it becomes clear that her posture of proud self-sufficiency is a defensive one, a stance that has protected her from having to feel the pain of her loneliness — and she begins to get in touch with the deep sadness within her about how alone she has always felt.

> **HOW DOES THE CONFLICT STATEMENT ATTEMPT TO KEEP THE CONFLICT WITHIN THE PATIENT INSTEAD OF BETWEEN PATIENT AND THERAPIST?**

The conflict statement highlights the tension within the patient between the healthy "Yes" forces and the unhealthy (resistive) "No" forces. Better that the conflict be within the patient than between patient and therapist.

The therapist wants to avoid being in the untenable position of "representing reality" or being the "voice of reality." When the therapist becomes the voice of reality, he is pitting himself against the patient and indirectly forcing the patient to protest ever more vehemently the legitimacy of the patient's defensive posture, ever more vehemently the legitimacy of his own convictions about reality.

By striving always to name what the patient knows to be real (and not what the therapist knows to be real), the therapist avoids engaging in battle with the patient. The therapist is, therefore, ever busy highlighting the conflict within the patient between what the patient knows he should feel/do and what the patient feels/does instead — which the therapist is able to do by way of conflict statements that juxtapose the patient's knowledge of reality with his experience of it.

If the therapist is the mouthpiece for what's right, healthy, and real, then it becomes unnecessary for the patient to access his own knowledge of what's right, healthy, and real. If the therapist takes responsibility for the patient's improvement (by speaking up on behalf of what the patient should do), then the therapist will be obviating the need for the patient to take responsibility for his own

RESPONDING TO THE PATIENT

forward movement. If the therapist carries the patient's hope (by believing in the patient and the patient's potential), then here too he may well be depriving the patient, ultimately, of the opportunity to access his own hope and belief in himself.

More generally, if the therapist is ever busy articulating the healthy side of the patient's conflict about improvement and change, then the patient may be stuck with speaking up on behalf of the unhealthy side of his conflict. If the therapist names what he thinks the patient should do in order to get better, then the patient is left with protesting his need to maintain the status quo.

But by way of statements that name the conflict as an internal one, the therapist avoids potential struggles with the patient in which he (the therapist) is the spokesperson for what the patient should be feeling and doing. In other words, better that the therapist say, "On some level, you know that if you are ever to get better, you will need someday to move beyond your anger at your father, but for now you are so enraged at him for all of what he's done to you that you can't imagine ever being able, really, to do that," than that the therapist say, "If you are ever to get better, you will need someday to move beyond your anger at your father."

In the first statement, the therapist is both locating the conflict within the patient (between what the patient knows he must eventually do and where he is in the moment) and articulating, on the patient's behalf, his understanding of why the patient might have trouble doing what the patient knows, eventually, he will have to do. In the second statement, the therapist not only fails to articulate his appreciation for how enraged the patient still feels but also, by simply telling the patient what the therapist thinks the patient should do, puts the patient on the defensive. In response to being told what he will have to do eventually, the patient may well protest that he is so enraged that he can't imagine ever being able to work through his anger with his father. The battleground, unfortunately, will now be between patient and therapist—not within the patient, which is where it should be.

As another example, consider the difference between "Although you know that if you are ever to recover custody of your kids you will need to make all sorts of changes in the way you live your life, in the moment you're not quite sure whether you'll really be able to make those changes or not" and "If you are ever to recover custody of your kids, you will need to make all sorts of changes in the way you live your life." Clearly, the patient will be able to hear more easily the first intervention (which articulates, in an experience-near fashion, the patient's conflict about changing) than the second (which simply tells the patient that she will have to change).

By way of conflict statements that strive to make the patient aware of the fact that there is conflict within him between the "forces of good" and the "forces of bad," the therapist locates the locus of the conflict within the patient—thereby furthering the patient's understanding of himself.

WHAT DOES A DEFENSE-AGAINST-AFFECT CONFLICT STATEMENT ADDRESS?

In the example above, of the therapist's informing the patient about his upcoming vacation, the therapist makes use of a defense-against-affect conflict statement to highlight what he senses it must have been like for his patient when she was young and was given full responsibility for the care of her little brother. He suspects that, as a child, she must indeed have felt abandoned and very much on her own—but that she could not bear to feel her loneliness and so defended herself against feeling that painful affect by clinging to her pride about being so responsible and able to handle whatever challenges might present themselves.

As we know, more generally, a patient is in conflict about many things. There is something that creates anxiety (about which the patient may be fully conscious, only dimly conscious, or completely unaware); there is also something that defends against that anxiety.

As we discussed earlier, the anxiety-provoking reality may be an intrapsychic reality, like an affect (as in the example above), or an interpersonal reality, something real about an object that makes the patient anxious—perhaps something disillusioning or something that challenges the patient's characteristic ways of experiencing himself and his objects.

For now, let us think about the situation that arises when the patient is resistant to acknowledging the presence of an anxiety-provoking affect, a situation that lends itself well to the therapist's formulation of a defense-against-affect conflict statement.

I will discuss such an intervention in some detail to demonstrate

RESPONDING TO THE PATIENT

more generally the ways in which conflict statements can be used, whether to highlight defenses against anxiety-provoking intrapsychic realities (as this defense-against-affect conflict statement does) or to highlight defenses against anxiety-provoking interpersonal realities (as do many of the conflict statements discussed later).

The defense-against-affect conflict statement is an attempt by the therapist to articulate, in a way that will make sense to the patient, the conflict the therapist senses the patient is having around allowing himself to experience an intolerable affect.

In making the statement, the therapist attempts to engage both the patient's experiencing ego and his observing ego; the therapist wants both to validate the patient's experience and to enhance the patient's knowledge. To that end, the therapist both resonates with where he senses the patient is (thus providing validation) and articulates, on the patient's behalf, his understanding of the conflict with which the patient is struggling (thus enhancing the patient's knowledge of himself and his internal process). The goal is to make the patient ever more aware of the tension within him between the affect he defends himself against and the defense that protects him from having to feel it.

WHAT ARE EXAMPLES OF DEFENSE-AGAINST-AFFECT CONFLICT STATEMENTS?

"You know that you are sad, but you are determined not to cry."

"You know that there is a reservoir of tears inside, but you are afraid that if you were ever to start crying, you might never stop."

"It upsets you when we talk about the problem you have managing your time, but you don't like to let that show."

"You know that you are sad, but it's hard to let yourself shed tears when you are remembering that your father used to tell you that only sissies cried."

"Even though you recognize that you must be sad, it is hard for you to let yourself feel it fully."

"You are concerned about how tired you have been feeling, but it upsets you to think that there might be something wrong with you."

"You are disappointed that you have not made more progress here, but you tell yourself that perhaps you were expecting too much."

"You know that you are disappointed, but you tell yourself that you have no right to be."

"You are upset, but you are not convinced that talking about it will do any good anyway."

The therapist must be able to understand and name, in a profoundly respectful way, both the reality the patient defends himself against and the defense itself. The therapist needs to understand that the patient both does and does not feel sad, both does and does not feel upset, both does and does not feel concerned, and both does and does not feel disappointed.

The patient who protests that he does not know how he is feeling, does not know how he is feeling; and the therapist must be respectful of the patient's need not to know. In his eagerness to get to the underlying affect, the therapist often boxes the patient into a corner by encouraging him to acknowledge his true feelings. Repeatedly the therapist asks the patient how he is feeling, even though the patient is clearly conflicted about feeling anything and has signaled that to his therapist. Insisting that the patient talk about how he is really feeling defeats the purpose of getting the patient more in touch with his affect, because it makes the patient more defensive, more resistant.

As an example, a patient is having trouble acknowledging the existence of his anger toward his mother. If we encourage him to express his anger, he may well oppose us by protesting that he is not angry with her, that in fact he is grateful to her for the many good things she has done for him over the years. In other words, he gets defensive, the protesting of his gratitude a defense against the acknowledging of his anger.

On the other hand, if we can appreciate that of course he has many feelings about his mother and if we can help him express both sides of his conflicted feelings, both his gratitude and his anger, then we have freed him up to acknowledge and to explore the whole range of feelings he has toward his mother. And so we might say something like "Although there must be times when you find yourself feeling impatient with your mother and annoyed by all her demands, for the most part you are deeply grateful to her for all that she has done for you over the years."

We are understanding that, even as the patient is feeling resentment and anger toward his mother, he does also feel grateful to her for her years of self-sacrifice. His need (albeit a defensive one) is to see her as having been very generous to him over the years. There is no need for the therapist to rob the patient of his gratitude; the therapist must respect the patient's need to protest his gratitude, because it would make him too anxious, at this point, to acknowledge other (negative) feelings. It is for the therapist to be patient; there will be time enough for the patient to access his annoyance, impatience, and resentment.

WHAT DOES THE FIRST PART OF THE DEFENSE-AGAINST-AFFECT CONFLICT STATEMENT DO?

The first part of the defense-against-affect conflict statement addresses the side of the conflict with which the patient, for now, is less in touch and less comfortable. The first part addresses the side of the conflict the patient defends himself against — an affect that would arouse anxiety in the patient were he to be made aware of its existence. The affect is there but, for now, is defended against, and the patient has difficulty acknowledging its presence.

WHAT DOES THE SECOND PART OF THE DEFENSE-AGAINST-AFFECT CONFLICT STATEMENT DO?

The second part of the defense-against-affect conflict statement addresses the side of the conflict with which the patient, for now, is more in touch and more comfortable. The second part addresses the side of the conflict that does the defending; it speaks to the defensive stance or posture that the patient has adopted as a result of the operation of his defenses. This side has to do, therefore, with the patient's investment in staying as he is, in preserving things as they are. This is the side that is less conflicted, less anxiety-provoking.

The second part of the statement, in essence, names the patient's resistance, in an experience-near, nonjudgmental fashion; it names the way the patient defends himself against having to experience his feelings.

WHY IS IT IMPORTANT THAT THE THERAPIST ADDRESS THE LEVEL OF THE PATIENT'S KNOWLEDGE OF HIS CONFLICT?

The therapist chooses his words carefully in order to make his interventions as experience-near as possible. To that end, it is important that he be ever attuned to the language the patient uses to describe his experience of things and to the level of awareness that the patient has achieved about both the things that make him anxious and the defenses he uses to protect himself against feeling that anxiety. The therapist must be able to speak the language of the patient and be able to articulate, in the patient's words, the patient's conscious or preconscious experience of his internal dilemmas.

For the patient to be receptive to conflict statements about forces that he may not be entirely aware of, the therapist must therefore address the patient's conscious or preconscious experience of his conflict. The statement attempts to formulate, in an experience-near fashion, what the therapist senses is the patient's internal experience of his conflict.

Ultimately, the therapist wants both to broaden and to deepen the patient's understanding of his internal psychodynamics; to do that, the therapist starts at the surface (in terms of the patient's level of awareness) and works downward (toward material that the patient is less aware of). If the therapist does not use language that is familiar to the patient, he will make the patient more anxious and will have defeated the purpose of enhancing the patient's understanding of his internal process.

RESPONDING TO THE PATIENT

> **WHAT IS THE DIFFERENCE BETWEEN HIGHLIGHTING WHAT THE PATIENT IS FEELING AND HIGHLIGHTING WHAT THE PATIENT KNOWS HE IS FEELING?**

With respect to the first part of the defense-against-affect conflict statement and how it names the patient's affect, there will be times, for example, when the therapist chooses to say "You are sad . . ." and other times when the therapist deems it more useful to say "You know that you are sad . . ." Both convey about the same thing but have slightly different emphases.

In the second intervention, the emphasis is a little more on the patient's knowledge of what he is feeling than on his actual experience of it. The patient is being given permission to step back from his experience of sadness in the moment in order to observe the fact that he knows he is sad; paradoxically, when the therapist gives the patient a little more distance, the patient is then freed up to acknowledge an affect that he might not otherwise have felt comfortable acknowledging.

> **WHAT IS THE DIFFERENCE BETWEEN HIGHLIGHTING WHAT THE PATIENT IS FEELING AND HIGHLIGHTING WHAT THE PATIENT KNOWS HE MUST BE FEELING?**

Note also the distinction between "You are sad . . ." and "You know you must be sad . . ." Again, both statements address the patient's affect but in slightly different ways.

In the second intervention, the emphasis is more on what the patient knows he must be feeling than on his actual experience of it. The therapist is appreciating that the patient knows enough about himself to be knowing that, even though he doesn't really feel sad, on some level he has to be sad. By suggesting that the therapist knows that the patient knows that he must be sad, the therapist is giving the patient permission not to be actually feeling the sadness. Paradoxically, this too may eventually free the patient up to feel his sadness.

> **WHAT IS THE DIFFERENCE BETWEEN HIGHLIGHTING WHAT THE PATIENT IS FEELING AND HIGHLIGHTING WHAT THE PATIENT FINDS HIMSELF FEELING?**

As we know, the second part of the defense-against-affect conflict statement names the defense the patient uses in order not to feel the affect named in the first part. Here, too, there are different ways to highlight the fact of the defense.

The therapist has the option of saying, for example, either "... you are feeling that ..." or "... you find yourself feeling that ..."

In the second intervention, the construction suggests that the patient need not take full ownership of what he discovers is within him. The therapist appreciates that the patient may be somewhat reluctant to acknowledge the way he really feels; the patient, for example, may feel ashamed of the way he defends himself against knowing. By giving the patient permission to deny total responsibility for the defense, paradoxically, the therapist may then free up the patient enough that he will be able to admit to himself and to the therapist how he really feels.

> **FINALLY, WHAT IS THE DIFFERENCE BETWEEN HIGHLIGHTING WHAT THE PATIENT IS FEELING AND HIGHLIGHTING WHAT THE PATIENT TELLS HIMSELF HE FEELS?**

Note the distinction between "You know you are disappointed, but you do not feel that you have a right to be" and "You know you are disappointed, but you tell yourself that you do not have a right to be."

With respect to the first statement, the therapist appreciates that the patient is pretty comfortable with his feeling that he is not entitled to be disappointed. With respect to the second statement, the therapist understands that the patient is defending himself against acknowledging his disappointment—but with much greater difficulty. The therapist appreciates that the patient is disappointed but is struggling with whether it is or is not all right to be disappointed.

IN OTHER WORDS, HOW DOES THE THERAPIST MAKE HIS INTERVENTIONS EXPERIENCE-NEAR?

The therapist must have been able to enter so completely into the patient's internal world that he is able to understand these fine points. He uses his understanding of how the patient really experiences both the affect he defends himself against and what he uses as his defense in order to inform the interventions the therapist then makes.

In summary, the therapist, in order to make his interventions experience-near, must be ever attuned to how he uses words to express his appreciation for both how the patient feels and how the patient defends himself against feeling that way. There are subtle differences between (1) what the patient feels and what he knows he feels, (2) what the patient feels and what he knows he must be feeling, (3) what the patient (defensively) feels and what he finds himself feeling, and (4) what the patient (defensively) feels and what he tells himself he's feeling. The therapist must appreciate such nuances in order to convey to the patient his understanding of the patient and his conflict.

HOW DOES THE DEFENSE-AGAINST-AFFECT CONFLICT STATEMENT BOTH VALIDATE EXPERIENCE AND ENHANCE KNOWLEDGE?

The defense-against-affect conflict statement attempts to address both the patient's experiencing ego and his observing ego, in order to give the patient the opportunity both to acknowledge how he is really feeling (or knows he must be feeling) and to step back so he can observe himself and his internal process. In this way the therapist hopes both to validate the patient's experience and to enhance his self-knowledge.

HOW DO CONFLICT STATEMENTS, MORE GENERALLY, ATTEMPT TO EMPOWER, VALIDATE EXPERIENCE, AND ENHANCE KNOWLEDGE?

More generally, the conflict statement (of which the defense-against-affect conflict statement is a specific instance) is intended to empower the patient or, rather, to encourage the patient to own the power he already has; the therapist is subtly encouraging the patient to take ownership of his conflict and of the tension within him between feeling and not feeling, between doing the right thing and not doing it, between acknowledging reality and needing to defend against it.

The therapist is suggesting, indirectly, that the locus of responsibility is an internal one—something that the patient has ultimate control over. By so doing, the therapist is facilitating internalization of the conflict; the conflict should be not an external one between the patient and his objects (including the therapist) but rather an internal one, within the patient.

Also, by juxtaposing the two sides of the patient's conflict, the therapist is attempting to pique the curiosity of the patient's observing ego. The therapist is encouraging the patient to observe himself and to recognize discrepancies between his knowledge of reality and his experience of it. Ultimately, the therapist is striving to create tension within the patient between what he knows to be real and what he experiences as real—tension that will eventually provide the impetus for change.

WHAT IS THE STRUCTURE OF THE CONFLICT STATEMENT?

"Although you know that . . . , nonetheless you feel that . . . "

"Although you know that you could do things differently if you really wanted to, in the moment it doesn't feel as if you have much control over what happens."

"Even though you know that you are disappointed in me and that

RESPONDING TO THE PATIENT

you will not be able to get beyond that until you have let yourself feel it, when you're feeling this despairing, it's hard to believe that anything could make any difference."

"Even though you know that you will need, eventually, to come to terms with just how angry you are with me, you would like to believe that you could get better without doing that."

"You know, on some level, that you have some control over what happens to you in the long run; but, on a day-to-day basis, it doesn't really feel that way."

"Even though you know that eventually you may have to leave him, at this point you are not yet prepared to do that."

"Even though you know that you could ask your parents for the money so that you would be able to continue your therapy, you are choosing not to because you do not want to be in the position of owing them anything."

"You know that you have paid a big price for having had parents who were always critical of everything you did, but you are hoping that you will be able to get better without having to get back into all that."

The therapist is ever busy naming, in an experience-near, nonjudgmental fashion, the ways in which the patient misperceives reality. In a conflict statement, the therapist juxtaposes the patient's knowledge of reality with his experience of reality. The therapist wants the patient to own his conflict, to own that he is conflicted. The therapist does not want to be the voice of reality that challenges the patient's ways of experiencing himself and his world of objects; rather, the therapist wants the patient to find that voice of reality within himself, to acknowledge what he (the patient) really does know to be real, even if sometimes he chooses to forget.

WHAT STANCE DOES THE THERAPIST TAKE IN RELATION TO THE PATIENT'S CONFLICT?

The therapist enters so completely into the patient's internal experience that he is able to understand both what the patient knows of the truth and how he defends himself against facing it.

In a conflict statement the therapist then articulates, on behalf of the patient, his understanding of the conflict with which the patient is struggling. The therapist does not pass judgment on the patient; he simply names what he senses is going on within the patient. He attempts to convey to the patient his respect for, and his deep appreciation of, the difficult choices the patient confronts. The therapist is not forcing the patient to take a stand, either to defend his current stance or to protest his wish to change.

HOW DO WE CONVEY OUR UNDERSTANDING OF A PATIENT'S INVESTMENT IN AN ABUSIVE RELATIONSHIP?

Let us consider a patient who cannot get out of an abusive relationship with his girlfriend. By way of listening very carefully, we come to appreciate that his need to stay in the relationship has to do with his feeling that although his girlfriend hurts him a lot, when she is good to him she makes him feel very special. And so we say to him:

"Although there must be times when you wonder why you don't just leave her, you can't bear the thought of not having her in your life because she makes you feel special and loved in a way that you have never before felt."

"Even though it bothers you when she treats you the way she does, you love her so much that you cannot imagine leaving her."

"Even though you hate it when she hurts you, you also know that no woman has ever made you this happy before."

We understand that the patient feels uneasy about the unhealthy relationship he has with his abusive girlfriend, but we also appreciate that he is so invested in the relationship that he is not about to give it up.

We must not need him to end the relationship with her because that's what we would do and think he should do. We must appreciate that, for the moment, the patient cannot leave the relationship

RESPONDING TO THE PATIENT 125

because it is still serving him in some way. The patient will not be able to leave his girlfriend until he has come to understand both what his investment is in staying and the price he pays for remaining in the relationship.

HOW DO WE HOPE THE PATIENT WILL RESPOND TO A CONFLICT STATEMENT?

By juxtaposing the force that says "Yes" and the counterforce that says "No," we are offering the patient an opportunity to elaborate upon either his investment in feeling/doing the things that would constitute mental health or his investment in feeling/doing the things that constitute his pathology. Now we are speaking not just to the conflict within the patient between feeling and not feeling but, more generally, to the conflict within the patient between his knowledge of reality and his experience of it (in other words, the conflict within him between his ability to perceive reality as it is and his need for illusion and distortion).

In response to a conflict statement, the patient either can go on to elaborate upon what he knows to be right (whether a feeling, an action, or a perception) or can explore his investment in maintaining things as they are. Our hope is that he will be stimulated to elaborate, in the form of associations, upon either his wish to get better or his need to remain the same.

As the patient explores, in ever greater depth, both sides of his conflict about change, he will begin to produce genetic material—to unearth significant events from his past and to revive childhood memories. As he begins to remember and reconstruct, patient and therapist begin to understand much better why and how the patient has come to be as he is.

In the example above, as the young man talks about how special he sometimes feels when he is with his girlfriend, he goes on to associate to how he never felt special growing up, that his mother was too wrapped up in other things to have much time for him, and that he grew up feeling very lonely and fearing that he would never find anyone to love him. He cries as he remembers just how unloved he had felt as a young boy; all the old pain is reawakened, the pain of his loneliness revived.

But he goes on to assert, with some indignation, that he is not sure how much longer he can stand being treated as shabbily as he is sometimes treated by his girlfriend. It does make him angry, and there are times when he thinks about leaving her. He starts to talk about how he would like to find someone who would be good to him all the time, someone whom he could really love and who would really love him.

He acknowledges that he had never imagined that he would be worthy of such love, because his experiences early on (in relation to his unavailable mother) had led him to believe that he would never find anybody who would pay attention to him and would want him in her life. He goes on to say that he is beginning to feel hopeful, that it may not have to be as it has always been, that he may yet be able to find the love for which he has been looking all his life.

WHAT ARE THE REALITIES AGAINST WHICH THE PATIENT FEELS THE NEED TO DEFEND HIMSELF?

I would suggest that we think, more generally, in terms of three different kinds of anxiety-provoking or painful realities against which the patient feels a need to protect himself: the reality that the patient needs eventually to confront, the price that he pays for refusing to confront that reality, and/or the grief work that he must ultimately do before he can get on with the therapy and his life.

WHAT ARE THE THREE DIFFERENT KINDS OF CONFLICT STATEMENTS CORRESPONDING TO THESE REALITIES?

Defense-against-reality conflict statements (which I will refer to, simply, as conflict statements) address themselves to anxiety-provoking or painful realities that will need eventually to be confronted. The defense-against-affect conflict statement discussed earlier is included in this category.

Price-paid conflict statements address themselves to the price that the patient pays for maintaining things as they are, by refusing to confront certain realities.

RESPONDING TO THE PATIENT

Work-to-be-done conflict statements spell out the grief work that the patient must ultimately do before he will be able to let go of his infantile attachments and his compulsive repetitions — in order to get on with his life.

In the first part of the conflict statement, then, the therapist gently confronts the patient's resistance by highlighting any of the following:

1. the reality (or affect) that the patient needs eventually to confront,
2. the price that he pays for refusing to confront that reality, and/or
3. the grief work that he must ultimately do before he can move forward.

In the second part of the conflict statement, the therapist eases up a bit by coming down on the side of the patient's resistance. The therapist highlights both intrapsychic and interpersonal defenses — in other words, both the defenses the ego mobilizes against the id and the defenses the self mobilizes against its objects.

These interpersonal defenses include the distortions, the illusions, and the entitlement that the patient clings to in order not to have to face the truth (both toxic and nontoxic) about his objects — namely, that they are other than who he had needed them to be.

MORE SPECIFICALLY, WHAT DOES A PRICE-PAID CONFLICT STATEMENT ADDRESS?

A price-paid conflict statement is a particular kind of conflict statement in which the therapist first names the price that the patient pays for maintaining the status quo of things (and refusing to confront certain realities) and then names the defense the patient uses to deny the price paid. A price-paid conflict statement is most effective when the patient has himself already begun to acknowledge that he pays some price for clinging to his old ways of feeling/doing. It is better that the patient be the one who begins to recognize the price he is paying for maintaining things as they are than that the therapist be the one who points it out to the patient.

Examples of price-paid conflict statements:

"Although you know that your reluctance to commit to the treatment makes our work more difficult, you find yourself holding back for fear of being hurt."

"Even though you know that your father's constant disapproval took its toll in terms of how you now feel about yourself, at this point you are hoping that you'll be able to get beyond it by trying really hard."

"You know that you do have a drinking problem and that you do things while under the influence that you later regret, but you tell yourself that you don't have to stop drinking entirely, what you do isn't that bad, and, anyway, you deserve to be able to be irresponsible sometimes."

"Even though you know that your bitterness has to do, in part, with things that happened to you early on, you are not yet prepared to confront those realities."

If the therapist senses that the patient has begun to see that there may be something problematic about how he has been living his life, something problematic about the ways in which he has been limiting both himself and his possibilities, the therapist may formulate a price-paid conflict statement in which he attempts to create further tension within the patient by emphasizing the cost to the patient of defending himself in the ways that he does. By so doing, he is able to direct the patient's attention to the price he pays for refusing to confront certain painful realities (past and present) in his life.

By way of such statements, the therapist strives to create tension within the patient so that it will be increasingly difficult for the patient to remain attached to his defense—in other words, so that the defense will become more ego-dystonic.

WHAT MUST THE PATIENT UNDERSTAND BEFORE HE CAN RELINQUISH THE DEFENSE?

Before the patient can relinquish a defense that he has clung to in order not to have to confront certain unbearably painful realities, he must come to appreciate (1) the fact that he is defended, (2) his

RESPONDING TO THE PATIENT 129

investment in the defense (in other words, how it serves him), and (3) the price he pays for holding on to it. He must come to understand, first, how his defenses protect him against the pain of knowing the truth about his objects and, then, how they ultimately create far more serious problems for him.

> **WHAT DOES A WORK-TO-BE-DONE CONFLICT STATEMENT ADDRESS?**

A work-to-be-done conflict statement is a particular kind of conflict statement in which the therapist spells out, in the first part of the statement, the work the patient must do before he can get beyond the place in which he is stuck and then, in the second part, names the defense that interferes with the patient's ability or willingness to do that work.

The therapist names for the patient the work the patient knows he must eventually do but then names, in a respectful manner, the forces the therapist believes are fueling the patient's resistance to doing that work. The patient can then go on either to explore what is involved in doing the work or to explore further the forces that interfere with his doing it.

Examples of work-to-be-done conflict statements:

"Even though you know that you will need, eventually, to come to terms with just how angry you are with me, you would like to believe that this too shall pass."

"You know that eventually, in order to overcome your fears about being close, you will have to let somebody in, but right now you're feeling that you simply cannot afford to take that risk."

"You know that, even though you have done some very good work to this point, there is still more work to be done, but at this point you are feeling that you have had enough."

"Even though you know that you are someday going to have to come to terms with just how disappointed you are in your mother, you find yourself thinking that it seems too overwhelming to get back into all that now and that maybe you'll be able to get better without having to do that."

"On some level you know that if you are ever to work all this through, you will need to let me be important to you, but at this point the thought of making yourself that vulnerable does not seem all that appealing."

In essence, the therapist is hoping to facilitate the working through of the patient's resistance by naming for the patient what the patient needs to do eventually in order to get better; the therapist makes a point of reminding the patient about realities that, for now, the patient defends himself against but that need ultimately to be confronted and mastered — and the patient knows it. It will be as the patient comes to terms with these realities and grieves them that, in time, he will get to a place where he can accept reality as it is, no longer needing it to be otherwise.

> **WHAT, MORE GENERALLY, DO CONFLICT STATEMENTS HIGHLIGHT?**

Conflict statements first highlight the thing that the patient is defending himself against: the reality that the patient needs to confront, the price that he pays for refusing to do so, and/or the grief work that he must ultimately do. Conflict statements then highlight the thing doing the defending: either an intrapsychic defense that the ego uses to protect itself against anxiety/pain or an interpersonal defense that the self uses to protect itself against anxiety/pain experienced at the hands of an object.

> **IN THE FOLLOWING CONFLICT STATEMENTS, WHAT DOES THE PATIENT DEFEND AGAINST AND WHAT IS DOING THE DEFENDING?**

"Even though you know that you are angry with me [reality], for now you don't want to think about it [defense]."

"Even though you know that you are holding back in here because you're so angry with me [reality, price paid], you're not yet willing to let go of that anger [defense]."

"Even though you know that you are disappointed in me and will not be able to get beyond that until you have let yourself feel the full range of feelings that you have about me right now [reality, price paid, work to be done], you would like to believe that this too shall pass [illusion]."

"Even though you know that you will need, eventually, to come to terms with just how angry you are with me [reality, work to be done], you would like to believe that you could get better without doing that [illusion]."

"Even though you know that your father was very mean to you [reality], you keep telling yourself that it must have been you who provoked it [distortion — burden of badness upon the self in order to preserve the illusion of the parent as good]."

"Even though you know that your father was very mean to you and that you've paid a steep price for that in terms of how you now feel about yourself [reality, price paid], for now you don't want to have to talk about it [defense]."

"Even though you know that you have some resentment toward your mother for having failed you in the ways that she did [reality], you tell yourself that you should be grateful to her for all the sacrifices she has made on your behalf over the years [defense — reaction formation]."

"Even though you know that your father was mean to you and that someday you're going to have to let yourself get in touch with just how enraged you are about that [reality, work to be done], it's easier to think of yourself as undeserving than to face how limited he was [distortion]."

"Even though you know that you're in a rage at your mother because of how unsupportive she was [reality], nonetheless you find yourself forgiving her because you feel that, under the circumstances, she did the best she could [defense — rationalization]."

"Even though you are beginning to understand that you may not always be able to have it on your terms [reality], you are not yet ready to give up wanting it that way [entitlement]."

"Even though you know that someday you're going to have to face all the feelings that you have about your mother [reality, work to be done], for now you are more inclined to take it out on yourself in the form of all sorts of self-destructive behaviors than to deal with just how enraged you really are with her [defense — acting out instead of sitting with]."

"Even though you know that you are someday going to have to recognize that your mother was never there for you in the ways that you would have wanted [reality, work to be done], you find yourself thinking that if she could but admit that she was wrong, then it would make things so much easier [illusion]."

"Even though you know that you will never really be able to be your own person until you can face the reality that no matter what you do it will never be good enough for your father [reality, price paid, work to be done], for now you are convinced that if you could but get him to see how successful you've become, then all would be well [illusion]."

"Even though you know that you won't get better until you make a commitment to coming regularly to the therapy [reality, price paid, work to be done], you resent having to pay and feel that you shouldn't have to come [entitlement]."

HOW DOES A CONFLICT STATEMENT BOTH CONFRONT THE PATIENT AND PARADOX HIM?

A conflict statement, whatever its kind, can be used either to confront or to paradox.

If the therapist chooses to emphasize an anxiety-provoking reality that the patient would really rather not feel (or know), then the therapist is in the position of confronting the patient. If the therapist chooses instead to stress the anxiety-assuaging defense to which the patient clings in order not to feel (or know), then the therapist may end up paradoxing the patient.

The therapist decides where to put the emphasis based on his sense of what the patient, in the moment, most needs and/or can tolerate.

WHAT ARE EXAMPLES OF CONFLICT STATEMENTS THAT CONFRONT?

"Even though you know that on some level you are absolutely enraged with me, you are not yet willing to talk about that."

"Although you know that, before you can let yourself get close to another man, you will have to work through your relationship with your ex-husband, you are not yet prepared to let go of your anger about how it ended."

"Even though you know that someday you will have to deal with these issues before you can have the quality of life that you seek, for now you are feeling that you have done what you can."

In these examples, the therapist is coming down solidly on the side of the force that needs eventually to be acknowledged, confronted, worked through, and mastered. The therapist recognizes that, in so doing, he is increasing the patient's anxiety, but there will be times when the therapist deems it appropriate and even advisable to do just that.

WHAT ARE EXAMPLES OF CONFLICT STATEMENTS THAT PARADOX?

"Although you sometimes find yourself resenting the weekly visit to your mother in the nursing home, you tell yourself that, after all she's done for you in her time, the weekly visit is the least you can do to show her how deeply grateful you are."

"Even though it means sometimes that you have to neglect your own needs, it feels so good to know that you are being helpful to others that it is well worth whatever suffering you might have to endure. No price is too great if it means being able to ease someone else's pain."

In these examples, the therapist is coming down so solidly on the side of the patient's defense that, in effect, the therapist is paradoxing the patient.

In the first example, the therapist is even insinuating that the patient's weekly visit to the nursing home (which the therapist recognizes is a piece of the patient's defensive need to protest his love and gratitude) may not even be enough! The patient, in response to the therapist's paradox, may actually counter the therapist's move with a heartfelt insistence that he feels his weekly visit is more than enough — in fact, perhaps more generous than is even necessary. By way of this paradox, the therapist may enable the patient to access his anger with his mother for how demanding she is of him and his time. By speaking up on behalf of the patient's guilt, the therapist will have forced the patient to speak up on behalf of his own needs.

In the second example, the therapist is so completely joining the patient's defensive need to sacrifice and suffer for the sake of others, whatever the cost, that the therapist may well force the patient to protest that there are limits to what he is willing to do for the sake of others. By forcefully reinforcing the patient's self-sacrifice, the therapist will have enabled the patient to get in touch with the healthy part of him that appreciates the need to take care of himself and his own needs.

HOW DOES THE THERAPIST TITRATE THE PATIENT'S ANXIETY?

When the therapist addresses both sides of the patient's conflict — that is, both those forces that provoke the patient's anxiety and those forces that ease it — he is able to modulate the level of the patient's anxiety. First the therapist increases the patient's anxiety by directing the patient's attention to something the patient would rather he didn't and then, just as the patient is beginning to feel anxious and therefore defensive, the therapist comes down on the side of the patient's defense by being with the patient where he is — which eases the patient's anxiety and makes him less defensive.

WHAT IS THE OPTIMAL LEVEL OF ANXIETY?

At any given point in time and for each patient, there is an optimal level of anxiety. Too little produces no impetus for movement of any kind, whereas too much produces immobilization and leads to an intensification of the patient's defensive efforts. By emphasizing either the ego-dystonic aspects of the patient's conflict (in the first part of the conflict statement) or the ego-syntonic aspects (in the second part), the therapist is able either to increase or to decrease the level of the patient's anxiety.

The optimal level of anxiety depends on many things — how motivated the patient is to get better, how interested he is in gaining insight, the depth of understanding he has acquired about his conflict, his degree of ego strength, and how solid the therapeutic alliance is, to name a few. From moment to moment, the therapist uses his intuition to assess just what that optimal level is.

Early on in the treatment, the patient may well be more invested in preserving the status quo than in changing. Consequently, the more anxiety-provoking side of the patient's conflict (his wish to change) is put in the first part of the conflict statement, and the less anxiety-provoking side (his resistance to change) is put in the second part.

Later on, as the patient comes to understand both his investment in the defense and the price he pays for maintaining that investment, it may come to pass that it creates more anxiety to be reminded of his resistance to change than to be reminded of his wish to change.

WHAT IS AN INVERTED CONFLICT STATEMENT?

An inverted conflict statement, which at this point may be more useful to the patient, is a statement in which the therapist intuitively inverts the order in which he names the two sides of the patient's conflict. Whereas a conflict statement speaks first to the patient's health (his wish to change) and then to his pathology (his resistance to change), an inverted conflict statement speaks first to his pathology and then to his health.

Note the difference between "Even though you know that you must someday deal with just how angry you get, at this point you are not quite yet prepared to do that" and "At this point you are not quite yet prepared to deal with just how angry you get, but you do know that you will someday have to deal with that."

The first, a conflict statement, emphasizes the patient's defensive need to wait until he's ready before he does the work he knows he must do. The second, an inverted conflict statement, emphasizes the patient's recognition that he does know there is work to be done (even if he is not quite yet prepared to commit to doing it).

The inverted conflict statement is clearly addressed to a patient who is getting more and more ready to do the work he knows he must do — namely, to understand why he has such a short fuse. Whereas once it made him anxious to think about doing the work and eased his anxiety when he reminded himself that he was not yet prepared to do it, now it makes him anxious to think about delaying indefinitely and eases him anxiety when he thinks about coming to grips with why he always gets so angry. Whereas once the defense — the self-protective need to delay the work to be done — was ego-syntonic (that is, eased his anxiety), now the defense is becoming increasingly ego-dystonic.

More generally, as the patient gets more and more in touch with the price he pays for feeling/doing as he does, as he begins to recognize the self-imposed limitations on his functioning because of his investment in maintaining things as they have always been, and as he begins to experience more and more acutely the pain he feels because of some of the choices he has made, the therapist may find himself intuitively inverting the conflict statement, so that now the first part of the statement addresses the patient's resistance to change and the second part addresses the patient's wish to change.

At the point when it becomes more anxiety-provoking for the patient to hold on to his defense than to confront the reality he has been defending himself against, then the patient will be forced to relinquish the defense. At this point, the patient's conflict with respect to the particular issue at hand will have been resolved, this piece of the resistance overcome, and the patient more able to move forward in the treatment and in his life.

TO WHAT EXTENT DOES THE THERAPIST CONFRONT THE DEFENSE, SUPPORT THE DEFENSE, OR DO BOTH?

We have suggested that in situations of conflict, the therapist has the option of (1) challenging the patient's defense by naming the anxiety-provoking reality the patient is defending himself against; (2) supporting the patient's defense by highlighting its existence in an experience-near, nonjudgmental, nonconfrontative fashion; or (3) first challenging the defense and then, just as the patient is feeling anxious, coming down on the side of the defense in order to support it.

To what extent does the therapist challenge, to what extent support, and to what extent do both? Each therapist has a different therapeutic style. Some therapists prefer to move in close to the patient in order to confront him — even if it means making the patient very anxious. Some therapists, however, prefer a more validating, less confrontative approach; they maintain more distance, respecting the patient's need to pace himself. Finally, some therapists prefer to create tension within the patient by repeatedly offering statements that first direct the patient's attention to where the therapist would like the patient to be and then resonate with where the patient is.

Although I have dwelled extensively on conflict statements, I am not suggesting that they be used exclusively. I have presented my ideas about conflict statements (and their various uses) because they demonstrate so clearly the ways in which the therapist can titrate the level of the patient's anxiety in order to be maximally effective.

It is crucial that the therapist be ever attuned, on a moment-by-moment basis, to the patient's capacity to tolerate anxiety and/or painful affect. When the therapist is able to keep in mind the delicate balance between the patient's capacity to feel/know and his need to defend against feeling/knowing, then conflict statements (by juxtaposing the patient's knowledge of reality with his experience of it) can be extremely effective tools for creating a state of dynamic tension within the patient, a fulcrum for eventual change.

WHAT IS YOUR OWN STYLISTIC PREFERENCE?

In my own practice, most of my interventions support the patient's defense by going with the resistance. Then, when the moment feels intuitively right, I will challenge the patient's defense — by reminding him of something that he really does know, even if sometimes he chooses to forget it. For the most part, then, I validate the patient's experience by being with him where he is; but, in those usually rare moments when I sense that there is a window of opportunity, I will attempt to enhance his knowledge of himself by directing his attention to something he has been defending himself against.

If the patient is made anxious by my confrontation and the pendulum starts to swing back toward defense, then I may choose to offer the patient a conflict statement that gently reminds the patient of the anxiety-provoking reality he is fleeing from and then resonates with the defensive posture he has assumed in order to restore his internal equilibrium. He can then choose to elaborate upon either the reality he is defending himself against or his need for the defense.

I also use conflict statements when I sense that the patient has the capacity to engage both his observing ego and his experiencing ego, has the capacity to hold in mind simultaneously both his knowledge of reality and his experience of it — and can profit from that juxtaposition.

FOR CONFLICT STATEMENTS TO BE EFFECTIVE, WHAT CAPACITIES MUST THE PATIENT HAVE?

As we know, a conflict statement highlights both what the patient knows and what the patient experiences. For the patient to be able to make good use of a conflict statement, therefore, he must have the capacity to experience two (disparate) things at the same time. If he cannot simultaneously hold in mind two different things, then he will be unable to make use of conflict statements. In other words, if he has no capacity to experience internal conflict, then he will not profit from the therapist's use of statements that locate, within the patient, conflict between two opposing forces.

Patients who cannot hold in mind simultaneously two different things in conflict with each other will tend to externalize. From this it follows that patients who tend to externalize may find it particularly difficult to be in the position of having to take responsibility for their conflict — because they do not have the capacity to recognize that the locus of their conflict is an internal, not an external, one.

Or if the patient does not have the capacity to sit with internal conflict and, instead, has the need to act it out, then the therapist's conflict statements will fall on deaf ears.

Finally, for a conflict statement to be effective, the patient must have some ability to acknowledge reality; he must be able to acknowledge that at least a part of him really does know what's real, what's right, what's healthy. Otherwise, the patient will have no use for an intervention that requires of him that he be able to admit that he has some awareness of what he should be feeling/doing.

> **WHAT IS THE CLASSIC EXAMPLE OF A PATIENT WHO LACKS THE CAPACITY TO TOLERATE INTERNAL CONFLICT?**

The borderline personality is, of course, the classic example of a patient who cannot tolerate internal conflict and, instead, acts it out. Because such patients have a tenuously established libidinal object constancy at best, they are unable to hold in mind simultaneously two sides of anything, including conflict. In fact, the hallmark of a borderline is that he lacks the capacity to sit with internal conflict and intense affect (particularly rageful disappointment) and, instead, tends to act it out in impulsive, destructive ways; he truly cannot contain himself.

The borderline's difficulty remembering the good in the face of the current bad (because of his inability to hold in mind both the good and the bad) makes it hard for him to master disappointment.

To master disappointment, a patient must be able to remember the good that had been there prior to the introduction of the bad. It is this capacity to remember that enables him to tolerate empathic failure, to tolerate disillusionment; it is this capacity to hold in mind simultaneously both the good and the bad that enables the patient to process and ultimately to master disappointment. He can then internalize the good that had been and, in the process, build up internal structure (in the form of further capacity) — optimal disillusionment and transmuting internalization.

The borderline, however, lacking libidinal object constancy, has not yet achieved the capacity to experience optimal disillusionment. For him, every disappointment is a traumatic one because, in the moment of the object's failure of him, the object becomes all bad and there is no memory of the good that had been. As a result, the disappointment cannot really be worked through and mastered. There is no taking in of the good and no building up of internal structure. The borderline, therefore, has neither the capacity to grieve nor the capacity to forgive. This also accounts for the borderline's notoriously defective capacity to internalize good things from the outside.

INSTEAD OF HELP WITH WORKING THROUGH CONFLICT, WHAT DOES THE BORDERLINE MOST NEED FROM THE THERAPIST?

Because the borderline cannot hold in mind simultaneously both his knowledge of reality and his experience of it, the mere naming of conflict will do little either to enhance the patient's knowledge or to validate his experience. What such a patient most needs is the provision of containment of his impulse to act out. What he most needs, then, is not understanding but restraint.

The borderline's inability to provide containment for himself fuels his need for the therapist to provide it for him. The patient's deficit involves his inability to contain himself; the need, therefore, is for the therapist to provide containment on the patient's behalf. In essence, the deficit creates the need; the need is for the therapist to serve as a deterrent, as a lid for the patient's id.

The heart of treatment for the borderline, then, lies in the therapist's preservation of the relationship in the face of repeated traumatic failures. The therapist's provision of external containment enables the relationship to continue, despite the frequent storms and crises.

In the aftermath of a disappointment, the borderline is tempted to sever his tie to the disappointing object. His inability to sit with his disappointment and his sense of outrage and frustrated entitlement at having been failed by his object fuel his impulse to act out and to take flight from what has become an intolerably painful situation.

The therapist must do everything he can to keep the patient alive and in treatment.

WHAT IS A CONTAINING STATEMENT?

I would like to propose that the therapist use containing statements in situations of actual crisis or potential crisis. Such statements first resonate with the affect the patient is experiencing in the moment and then bring the patient up short by reminding him of some reality.

Examples of conflict statements:

"Perhaps you would wish that you could stay; but, as you know, our time is up and we do have to stop for today."

"You just can't get rid of this idea that when you feel hurt by me, you are allowed to retaliate, even though you know that such behaviors are destructive to our relationship and to the bond we have worked so hard to develop."

"You think all the time about killing yourself to ease the pain; but you and I both know that if you actually succeeded, your kids would never get over it and would never forgive you."

"When you get angry like this, you think about taking flight; but we both know that someday you're going to have to stop running."

"You're hating me right now and thinking about killing yourself or breaking off treatment; but you and I both know that if you are ever going to understand why you have such trouble getting close to people, then someday you're going to have to slow down and give yourself a chance to figure out what keeps going wrong for you in relationships."

In each such statement, the therapist first resonates with the patient's affect and then reminds him of something that really does matter to him, even if he is forgetting that in the moment.

HOW DOES A CONTAINING STATEMENT BRING THE PATIENT UP SHORT?

Whereas a conflict statement first confronts and then supports, a containing statement first supports and then confronts. Also, whereas a conflict statement first directs the patient's attention elsewhere and then resonates with where the patient is, a containing statement first resonates with where the patient is (in order to engage the patient) and then directs the patient's attention to something that the therapist hopes will serve as a deterrent to the patient's acting out. In other words, by way of containing statements, the therapist must first get the patient's attention by resonating with where the patient is; then the therapist must bring the patient up short by directing the patient's attention to some reality that the therapist hopes will serve as a deterrent to the patient's temptation to act out. Although the patient may have lost sight of this reality in the moment, once he is reminded of it the patient can no longer continue to deny it.

The most effective containing statements are those that hook the patient because they address something that really does matter to him. For example, by reminding a patient who is very much invested in being a good mother that she will do irreparable damage to her children if she actually kills herself, the therapist may be able to serve, rather effectively, as a deterrent.

In short, the therapist must function as an external container because the patient lacks the capacity to provide this containment internally. It is the therapist's external provision of this containment that enables the patient to survive the crisis and to recover his capacity to behave more responsibly.

HOW, THEN, DO CONFLICT STATEMENTS FACILITATE THE PATIENT'S PROGRESS IN THE TREATMENT?

When the patient has an impaired capacity to tolerate internal conflict and is at risk for acting out, the therapist may not be able to formulate effective conflict statements because the patient does not have the ability to acknowledge that the responsibility for his actions is his own.

But when the patient has the capacity to sit with internal conflict and is not at risk for acting it out, the therapist is able to use conflict statements to facilitate the patient's progress in the treatment. In such statements, the therapist attempts to enhance the patient's knowledge by confronting him with what he really does know to be real, even if sometimes he would rather forget.

Although the therapist then goes on to relieve the patient's anxiety by supporting the defense that the patient mobilizes self-protectively, the therapist has had the opportunity to name a reality the patient has been busy defending himself against. The therapist is striving to put a wedge between the patient's knowledge of reality and his experience of it, in order to create tension within the patient that will ultimately provide the impetus for forward movement. As we know, as the defense becomes increasingly ego-dystonic, it becomes more and more necessary for the patient to relinquish it.

WHAT IS A PATH-OF-LEAST-RESISTANCE STATEMENT?

Let us look at two specific conflict statements:

"Even though you recognize that you may also be hurt, your experience is that you are simply angry."

"Although you know that there are some things you could do to make yourself feel better, you tell yourself that none of those things would make a real difference anyway."

In the first of these statements, the patient's conflict is between acknowledging how hurt he is, which is difficult to do because it makes him so anxious, and feeling his anger, which is a defense against the disappointment. In the second statement, the patient's conflict is between acknowledging that he is master of his own destiny, acknowledgment of which makes him anxious, and feeling that he is powerless, which is a defense against owning the responsibility he has for his life.

A conflict statement that highlights actual choices the patient has about how he lives his life lends itself nicely to being translated into a path-of-least-resistance statement, in which the therapist highlights the fact that it is easier for the patient to do what is old and familiar (which fuels his defense) — even if pathological — than for the patient to do something new, different, and more healthy. Such statements are in the nature of a confrontation and can be used to highlight the fact that the patient has a choice between two alternatives; by way of path-of-least-resistance statements, the therapist is encouraging the patient to take ownership of the decisions he makes.

The prototypical path-of-least-resistance statement first names the defense and then names the healthy force defended against:

"It is easier to . . . than to . . ."

In the examples that follow, the first statement in each pair is a conflict statement; the second is the path-of-least-resistance statement derived from it.

1. "Even though you recognize that you may also be hurt, your experience is that you are simply angry."
2. "It is easier to be angry than to acknowledge how hurt you must also be."

1. "Although you know that there are some things you could do to make yourself feel better, you tell yourself that none of those things would make a real difference anyway."
2. "It is easier to tell yourself that there is nothing you could do that would make a real difference anyway than to admit that there might be some things you could do to make yourself feel better."

1. "Even though you know that you should sit with just how ragefully disappointed you feel, a part of you is tempted to act it out."
2. "It is easier to act out your rageful disappointment than to sit with just how devastated you feel."

1. "Although you recognize you could have done things differently, you find yourself wanting to blame everyone else."
2. "It is easier to blame everyone else than to look at how you might have done things differently."

1. "Although you know that you could try to talk about just how upset you are, it is hard not to retreat."
2. "It is easier to retreat than to talk about just how upset you are."

1. "Even though you know that you do have choices, you find yourself feeling hopeless and helpless."
2. "It is easier to feel hopeless and helpless than to think about the choices you have."

In a path-of-least-resistance statement, the therapist is being intentionally somewhat provocative, somewhat confrontative, by suggesting that the patient is responsible for the decisions he makes. The therapist is saying that the patient, as helpless and as out of control as he may sometimes feel, is nonetheless ever busy making choices.

Furthermore, the therapist is implying that the patient often opts for the path that seems to offer the least resistance because that route is easier. The message to the patient is that the locus of responsibility is an internal one over which the patient has ultimate control.

WHAT CREATES THERAPEUTIC IMPASSES?

Think about the situation that arises when the patient, convinced as he is that he is so damaged from way back that there is really nothing he can do now, and nothing he should have to do now, is waiting for the therapist to come through, and the therapist, convinced as he is that the impetus for change must come from the patient, is waiting for the patient to come through.

Therapeutic impasses arise in these stalemated situations, in which the patient is convinced that he has done everything he can do (and certainly everything he could possibly have been expected to do) and that it is now up to the therapist to do the rest. The patient may not always recognize that he has such expectations of the therapist but, when such expectations are present, the work of the therapy cannot proceed until they have been unearthed and, eventually, worked through.

Therefore, it is important that the therapist tease out what the patient's underlying expectations are about who should take responsibility for the therapeutic work and that the therapist make conscious the patient's unconscious assumptions—so that such feelings can be explored in greater depth and understood as forces opposing the work of the treatment. Unacknowledged, they powerfully fuel the resistance and impede the patient's progress in the therapy. It may seem that the patient is doing the work that needs to be done—but he is actually waiting, waiting for the therapist to do it.

Many treatments get bogged down because of the patient's conviction (1) that he is so damaged from long ago that he truly cannot be held accountable for his life; (2) that, at this point, it is up to someone else (the therapist) to do whatever must be done; and (3) that he (the patient) is entitled to such recompense.

WHAT IS AN EXAMPLE OF A THERAPEUTIC IMPASSE?

Let us think about the situation that arises sometimes at the beginning of a session, when the patient is sitting quietly, waiting for the therapist to begin, while the therapist is sitting quietly, waiting for the patient to begin. The patient thinks it should be the therapist's responsibility to start the session; the therapist thinks it should be the patient's responsibility.

To identify whatever unconscious assumptions are fueling the patient's resistance, the therapist may choose to explore (1) the patient's underlying distortions (by way of statements like "You're not sure you know where to begin"); (2) the patient's underlying illusions (by way of statements like "Perhaps you're hoping I will get us started"); or (3) the patient's underlying entitlement (by way of statements like "You're not sure you should have to be the one to start").

By way of these various interventions, the therapist is encouraging the patient to elaborate upon (1) his experience of himself as not able, as so damaged and impaired from early on that he simply cannot help himself because he truly does not know how; (2) his expectation that the therapist is someone who does know how and who could therefore do it for him, if the therapist were but willing; and (3) his belief that he is entitled to such assistance now because of what he didn't get back then.

But as long as the patient clings to his distortions (I can't), his illusions (you can), and his entitlement (you should), he will not get better and will remain stuck in the treatment.

WHAT KINDS OF INTERVENTIONS DO WE MAKE WHEN THERE IS A THERAPEUTIC IMPASSE?

Therapeutic impasses (fueled by the patient's sense of himself as not able, his experience of the therapist as able, and his conviction that this is his due) are so common that I have developed several interventions designed specifically to highlight the underlying distortions, illusions, and entitlement that interfere with the patient's

RESPONDING TO THE PATIENT

ability to take responsibility for the treatment and his life: the damaged-for-life statement (to highlight the distortions), the compensation statement (to highlight the illusions), and the entitlement statement (to highlight the entitlement).

WHAT IS A DAMAGED-FOR-LIFE STATEMENT?

The first intervention is something I refer to as a damaged-for-life statement. Such a statement articulates what the therapist perceives to be the patient's conviction about his own deficiencies and limitations, a conviction that the patient uses, perhaps unconsciously, to justify his refusal to take responsibility for his life. The therapist highlights the patient's distorted perception of himself as a helpless victim and as therefore unable to do anything to make his life better.

The patient may experience himself as having an inborn, constitutional flaw; as having been victimized by bad parenting early on; or, more generally, as having been always a victim of injustice, a victim of fate, a victim of unfortunate external circumstances. In any event, he has a distorted sense of himself as damaged and therefore as lacking certain capacities.

A damaged-for-life statement attempts to articulate some of the underlying distortions that the patient clings to as unconscious justification for his inability/unwillingness to hold himself accountable. In such a statement, the patient's fatalism is named; the therapist resonates with the patient's belief that (1) the die has been cast, (2) he is destined for life to suffer, and (3) there is really nothing he can do now in order to make the situation any better.

Examples of damaged-for-life statements:

"Deep within you, you feel such despair, because of things that happened to you early on, that you can't really imagine ever being able to do anything that would make any kind of difference."

"You feel that you were cheated and ripped off as a kid, and so it's hard to believe that anything could make that different now."

"Because you were so deprived as a child, you feel that you don't now really have the necessary tools to do your life properly."

"You feel so incapacitated, so impaired, so damaged, that it's hard to imagine how things could ever be any different."

"You are in such pain, want so desperately to be free of it, and feel that you would do anything to get better, but you can't figure out what it is that you could possibly do to change things."

In a damaged-for-life statement, the therapist highlights the patient's experience of damage done early on and then highlights the patient's experience of his disability now. In essence, the therapist is making explicit the patient's distorted sense of himself as a helpless victim and as therefore not responsible.

WHAT IS A COMPENSATION STATEMENT?

Many patients feel, on some level, that they become full only by way of input from the outside. Because of damage sustained early on at the hands of their parents, they are now limited in terms of their own resources and must therefore rely upon input from the outside to make up the difference. In a compensation statement, the therapist calls attention to the patient's wish to be compensated now for damage sustained early on; the therapist highlights the patient's illusions about being able to find someone who will be able to make up the difference to him.

Whereas a damaged-for-life statement underscores the patient's distortions, his misperceptions of himself as a helpless victim, a compensation statement underscores the patient's illusions about his objects as potential providers of magic, answers, love, reassurance — all sorts of restoratives that will heal him and rectify the damage done early on.

If the therapist is in collusion with the patient's belief that the patient will get better only by way of input from the outside, then it will be very difficult for the therapist to tolerate being in the position of breaking the patient's heart, which will happen once the patient discovers that the therapist is not able to make up the difference to him.

Examples of compensation statements:

"You are wishing that I could do something to ease your pain."
"You feel that you've already done about as much as you possibly can. At this point, you're hoping that someone else will be able to do whatever needs to be done."

RESPONDING TO THE PATIENT

"Because you feel so confused and so overwhelmed, you find yourself looking to others for direction and guidance."

"At this point, you would like me to tell you what to do and where to go from here."

"At times like this, when you're feeling completely burnt out and exhausted, you find yourself thinking that you'll never get better unless someone else is willing to help you out."

If the patient is to move forward in the treatment and in his life, he must eventually understand that what he is holding out for is illusory. By having his wish for sustenance from the outside made explicit, the patient must ultimately confront the truth—namely, that his wish to be healed by way of external provision is illusion, not reality.

WHAT IS AN ENTITLEMENT STATEMENT?

In an entitlement statement, the therapist makes it explicit that the patient not only wishes for input from the outside but also feels entitled to such input, feels that it is his due, his right, his privilege to have someone from the outside make up the difference to him. Because he feels so cheated from long ago, he believes that he is now entitled to compensation to make up for the early-on environmental deficiencies.

Examples of entitlement statements:

"You are feeling that you have worked hard in the treatment and have done everything that you could possibly do on your own; you are feeling that it's now my turn to do something."

"You are thinking that it is not unreasonable to be expecting that, at this point, I be willing to help you out."

"You are feeling that I should be able to offer you interpretations that will pull the material together for you."

"You are wanting me to do something in order to help you recover more of the memories. You are feeling that that's my job."

"Your mother demanded the world of you and gave you nothing in return; at this point, you're feeling that you will not be satisfied unless she can acknowledge that she was wrong and can offer you an apology."

It is crucial that the patient's underlying sense of entitlement be recognized and named. Many patients reach an impasse in their treatment because, deep within their souls, they harbor the conviction that they have gone both as far as they can and as far as they should have to; it is now up to someone else. They believe that, since it was not their fault then, it should not be their responsibility now; they believe that, because of damage sustained long ago, they are entitled to recompense in the here and now. An entitlement statement highlights the fact of the patient's entitlement and may also contextualize it as a reaction to early-on privation, deprivation, or insult.

In summary, the patient's distorted sense of himself as so damaged from way back that he is not now responsible, his illusory sense of his objects as able to compensate him now for the early-on damage, and his entitled sense of being owed that compensation must be uncovered and named — because they fuel the resistance and seriously interfere with the patient's forward movement in the treatment and in his life.

> **MORE GENERALLY, WHAT HAPPENS WHEN THE PATIENT'S DISTORTIONS, ILLUSIONS, AND ENTITLEMENT GET DELIVERED INTO THE RELATIONSHIP WITH THE THERAPIST?**

Even though on some level the patient knows better, the patient is nonetheless always misinterpreting the present, making assumptions about the present based on the past. Because of early-on traumatic parental failures, the patient now both desperately yearns to find the good parent he never had (illusion) — he feels entitled to find that good parent (entitlement) — and desperately fears that he will find, instead, the bad parent he did have (distortion). He is forever misunderstanding his present in terms of his unresolved past.

RESPONDING TO THE PATIENT

When such misperceptions are delivered into the patient-therapist relationship, they give rise to the transference, both the positive transference (fueled by the patient's wish for good) and the negative transference (fueled by the patient's fear of bad). The transference is the way the patient misinterprets the present.

It is by way of working through the transference (both the disrupted positive transference and the negative transference) that the patient's need for his objects to be other than who they are becomes transformed into the capacity to accept them as they are. It is in the context of the safety provided by the relationship with the therapist that the patient is able to do, at last, the remembering, the confronting, the reexperiencing, and the grieving he has spent a lifetime defending himself against. He grieves for the wounded child he once was and the wounded adult he has now become.

It is by way of this working-through process that the need to experience reality in ways determined by the past is transformed into a healthy capacity to experience reality as it is. Only as the patient grieves, doing now what he could not possibly do as a child, will he get better. Only as he grieves will he be able to let go of his relentless pursuit of infantile gratification (which fuels the positive transference) and his compulsive reenactments of his unresolved childhood dramas (which fuel the negative transference).

It will be by way of this working-through process that the transferential need to experience his objects as other than who they are will become transformed into a mature capacity to experience and to accept them as they are.

Transformation of need into capacity, energy into structure, is what enables the patient to relinquish his defenses and his need not to know. As he finally confronts the reality of the parental limitations, he lets go of the defenses around which the resistance has organized itself. As he gradually gives up his defenses and overcomes his resistance, he becomes freer to experience reality as it is, uncontaminated by his infantile wishes and fears.

To work through the transference, a wedge must ultimately be put between the patient's experience of reality (inaccurate perceptions based on the past) and his knowledge of reality (accurate perceptions based on the present). It will then be the internal tension created through the patient's awareness of that discrepancy that will provide, ultimately, the impetus for change.

As the patient becomes ever more aware of the discrepancy

between objective reality and his experience of it, the synthetic function of the ego will become ever more active in its efforts to reconcile the two elements in conflict — and the balance will shift in favor of reality. It is this synthetic function of the ego that will make necessary the letting go of the past, the renunciation of infantile attachments, and the giving up of the illusions and distortions to which the patient has clung since earliest childhood in order not to feel his pain.

To lay the groundwork for these transformations, the illusions and distortions that inform the transference must be uncovered and exposed to the light of day; the patient's ways of perceiving both himself and his objects (particularly the therapist) must be teased out and named, which illusion and distortion statements do.

WHAT IS AN ILLUSION STATEMENT?

Once the patient's illusions have been delivered into the treatment situation, a positive transference unfolds. When a positive transference is in place and the patient is experiencing the therapist as the perfect parent he never had, there is no need for the therapist to do any interpreting. He should simply allow the positive transference to be, recognizing that it is an important backdrop for what is to come.

When the inevitable disruption occurs, occasioned by the therapist's empathic failure of the patient, the patient must be given the opportunity to work through and master the resultant disillusionment.

The working-through process will be easier if the therapist, prior to the disillusionment, has already named, in an experience-near, noninterpretive fashion, the patient's underlying magical expectations with respect to the transference object. Underscoring the fact of such illusions (as soon as they arise) will facilitate the working through of the patient's eventual and inevitable disenchantment, when it turns out that the therapist is not as perfect as the patient would have wanted the therapist to be.

In other words, it will be easier for the patient to work through his disillusionment if, earlier, the patient's hopeful expectations with respect to the therapy and the therapist have already been spelled

RESPONDING TO THE PATIENT

out, in a nonshaming, nonjudgmental manner. Illusion statements do just that. The format of an illusion statement is as follows:

"You are wishing that _____."
"You so want _____."
"You are hoping that _____."

Examples of illusion statements:

"You are feeling that you have finally found the safe place you've been searching for all your life."
"You had never thought that you would be able to feel this understood."
"You had never imagined that you could feel this hopeful."
"You so want to be able to feel that I know and deeply accept you, for all of who you are."
"You are hoping that I will be able to give you answers that will enable you to make sense of all this."

In an illusion statement, the therapist highlights the fact of the patient's hope—illusory hope, as it happens, but this aspect is not specifically emphasized. The therapist wants the patient to be aware of the hopes, longings, and dreams that the patient brings to the therapy and to his relationship with the therapist. Acknowledgment of illusory hope will provide an important foundation for the patient's working through of his eventual, and inevitable, disillusionment.

HOW ARE ILLUSION STATEMENTS USED TO SUGGEST DISILLUSIONMENT?

In the illusion statements that follow, the element of future disillusionment is already being introduced:

"You had so hoped that you would be feeling better by now."
"It had felt so good to be feeling so understood in here."

"You had dreamed of being able to find someone who would really understand."

"You were so wanting to find in here the kind of acceptance that you had never been able to find elsewhere."

In these statements, the therapist is understanding that, for whatever the reason, the patient's good feelings are starting to slip away; the patient's hopes are beginning to fade.

WHAT IS A DISILLUSIONMENT STATEMENT?

The working-through process is a prolonged grieving process and one that can be facilitated by the use of a disillusionment statement.

The disillusionment statement has two parts. In the first part, the therapist highlights the patient's underlying illusions about the therapist's perfection; in the second part, the therapist empathically resonates with the patient's experience of disillusionment, disappointment at the discovery of the therapist's imperfection. More generally, the disillusionment statement highlights the discrepancy between the illusion of the object as infallible and the reality of the object as fallible. It is used to facilitate the patient's accessing of his grief about the limitations of his objects (whether present or past).

Examples of disillusionment statements:

"You had so hoped that you would be feeling better by now, and it upsets you terribly that you still feel so awful."

"It had felt so good to be feeling so understood in here, and now you're beginning to feel that I may not always understand as much as you had thought I could."

"You had so hoped that talking about all this would make things better, but you are still feeling terrible and that angers you."

"You had so hoped that I would be able to give you answers, and it angers you that I haven't done that."

"All you had wanted was a little advice, and it bothers you that I haven't offered you that."

In a disillusionment statement, the therapist both names the underlying illusions and resonates with the patient's experience of disillusionment, in an attempt to make it easier for the patient to gain access to his grief about the failures of his objects (both the nontraumatic failures of the transference object and the traumatic failures of the infantile object). In essence, it facilitates the working through of the disrupted positive transference; it helps the patient do the grieving he must eventually do in order to come to terms with reality as it is.

IS A DISILLUSIONMENT STATEMENT A PARTICULAR KIND OF CONFLICT STATEMENT?

A disillusionment statement is not a conflict statement, in that it does not first name a reality the patient defends himself against and then the defense itself. It is, rather, a particular kind of legitimization statement (which will be discussed later), in that it attempts to frame the patient's current experience of disillusionment as an understandable reaction to having had hopes that were crushed. Given that the patient had thought the therapist was (or, at least, would someday become) the perfect parent he had never had, of course the patient is now devastated by the therapist's demonstration of his fallibility.

WHAT IS AN INTEGRATION STATEMENT?

An integration statement can be used in the aftermath of empathic failures that have so devastated the patient that, in the moment, he can no longer remember whatever good there might have been prior to that moment. The therapist enters into the patient's internal experience of upset, outrage, and disillusionment and appreciates that, in the face of the current bad, memories of past good cannot be recovered.

An integration statement acknowledges the patient's difficulty holding on to good feelings when he is feeling angrily disappointed. In an integration statement, the therapist resonates with the patient's current feeling of disappointment and, by highlighting the patient's difficulty remembering past good in the face of his current upset, gently reminds the patient of his previous experience of having felt good. Integration statements are used to facilitate the patient's remembering.

By way of an integration statement, the therapist wants to help the patient hold in mind, simultaneously, both the good (that is, the past experience of having been gratified) and the bad (that is, his present experience of disillusionment and frustration). To that end, the integration statement (1) acknowledges the patient's current feeling of upset; (2) remembers for him the good he has forgotten; and (3) articulates, on his behalf, the difficulty he has remembering it.

Integration statements are particularly useful for borderlines, who, because of their tenuously established libidinal object constancy, have much difficulty holding in mind at the same time both good and bad. In the aftermath of a disappointment or frustration, the once good object becomes all bad, because the borderline, in the face of the present bad, cannot retain memories of the former good.

Examples of integration statements:

"When you are feeling this upset, it's difficult to remember the good times."

"When you're feeling this devastated, it's hard to remember that you used to feel good in here and looked forward to coming."

"When you are this angry, it's hard to recall ever having felt not angry."

"When your heart is hurting, as it is now, you can't remember ever having felt hopeful."

The following integration statements introduce the element of the patient's difficulty sustaining hope for the future in the light of his current upset, outrage, and despair:

"When your heart is breaking, as it is now, you can't imagine ever trusting me again."

"When you are this angry, you lose whatever good feelings you might have had about me and cannot imagine ever being able to recover them."

"When you are feeling this hurt by me, it is hard to believe that you will ever be able to recapture whatever good feelings you might once have had about me."

"When you are feeling this kind of despair, it feels as if your heart is breaking and won't ever be whole again."

In an integration statement, the therapist does not simply remind the patient of what the patient, on some level, does know — namely, that things were good once (and may become good at some point in the future). For example, the therapist does not simply tell the patient, "But you used to feel so good about me and our work together!" Such a blunt reminder by the therapist of something the distraught patient can no longer keep in mind may be experienced by the patient as a confrontation and may create the potential for a struggle between them.

More useful is an intervention in which the therapist, appreciating that the patient truly cannot, in the moment, remember the good that had been, resonates empathically with the patient's difficulty remembering that good: "When you're feeling this disappointed, it is hard to remember that you used to feel good about me and our work together."

In summary, integration statements are used to assist the patient's working through of his bad feelings about someone once experienced as good; they are useful adjuncts to disillusionment statements, both of which strive to facilitate the working through of the disrupted positive transference.

WHAT IS A DISTORTION STATEMENT?

Once the patient's distortions have been delivered into the treatment situation, a negative transference unfolds, in which the patient experiences the therapist as the bad parent he once had. When a negative transference is in place, the relationship with the therapist recreates the early-on traumatic relationship with the bad parent.

Whereas positive transferences need not be interpreted (only their disruptions), negative transferences must always be interpreted, because, as long as they go unchallenged, the patient's distorted perceptions of the therapist as the powerfully victimizing parent he once had and of himself as the powerless victim he once was will be reinforced—and the patient's forward movement in the treatment and in his life will be seriously compromised.

Until the negative transference has been worked through and resolved, the patient will be unable to use the transference object as a new good object. Furthermore, the negative transference must be interpreted if there is to be an opportunity for belated mastery, an opportunity both to rework the original traumas and to transform the internalized badness into healthy capacity.

To facilitate the eventual working through of the negative transference, the therapist wants to encourage the patient to observe the fact of his unconscious repetitions and to see that he does rather tend to make assumptions about present objects based upon negative experiences with past objects.

The therapist, therefore, offers the patient distortion statements that name, in an experience-near, nonchallenging fashion, the expectations the patient would seem to have about his current objects (including the therapist) based on his unresolved past.

Examples of distortion statements:

"You are assuming that I, like your mother, will be critical."

"Your fear is that I will turn out to be as relentlessly demanding as your father was."

"You are expecting me to be the same kind of dissatisfied with you that your mother was."

"You are afraid that I will betray you as you have been betrayed in the past."

"It is hard to imagine that someone might turn out to be different from the way everyone else has always been."

"You are feeling in here with me the same kind of helpless and victimized that you have always felt in the past."

"I too have now failed you as all those before me eventually failed you."

In a distortion statement, the therapist either implies or makes explicit a connection between the patient's current experience of the therapist as bad and the patient's early-on experience of the parent as bad; the therapist does not say that the patient's current perceptions are distorted, but he does encourage the patient to observe the fact of recurring themes, patterns, and repetitions in his life and in his relationships.

WHAT IS A LEGITIMIZATION STATEMENT?

Whereas illusion statements highlight underlying illusions and whereas distortion statements highlight underlying distortions, legitimization statements are used to highlight both illusions and distortions and to contextualize these unrealistic perceptions of reality as legitimate, reasonable responses to things that had come before.

The legitimization statement places into perspective, into historical context, both the unrealistically positive and the unrealistically negative misperceptions the patient has of the therapist (and of himself). It is used when the therapist wants both to enhance the patient's knowledge of why he has come to believe as he does about himself and his objects and to convey empathically to the patient that the therapist understands why the patient believes as he does.

The prototypical legitimization statement first names the historical antecedent and then names the result:

"Given that . . . then, of course . . . now."

Such an intervention suggests that, given the nature of his past, of course now the patient has both certain wishes and certain fears. A legitimization statement validates the patient's current wishes and fears, suggests that, in the light of his past, it is entirely understandable that the patient would have come to be as he is and to feel as he does. In other words, it stresses the genetic underpinnings of the patient's current defensive stance, contextualizing it as a derivative of early-on bad experiences.

In the following examples, the first legitimization statement in each pair highlights the patient's wish, his hope that things will be different this time; the second statement highlights his fear that they won't:

1. "Given that your mother was so reluctant to give you approval, of course now you find yourself hoping that you'll be able to get that from me."
2. "Given that your mother was so reluctant to give you ap-

proval, of course now you find yourself fearing that you won't be able to get that from me either."

1. "Given that you were so misunderstood by your parents, of course now you are desperately hoping to find the understanding you've been seeking for so long."
2. "Given that you were so misunderstood by your parents, of course now you are terribly afraid that you'll be misunderstood by me too."

1. "Given that you never felt special as a child, of course you would want to be able to know that you are special here."
2. "Given that you never felt special as a child, of course your fear is that here too your heart will be broken."

Legitimization statements are useful for contextualizing both the illusions that accompany the positive transference and the distortions that accompany the negative transference. All such statements validate or legitimize the patient's current feelings of yearning, desire, vulnerability, susceptibility, anxiety, insecurity, fearfulness, or dread as derivatives of early-on traumatogenic experiences with the parent.

We may even formulate a statement that legitimizes both wish and fear:

"Because you had no one you could depend upon as you were growing up, of course now you find yourself wanting to be able to depend upon me but wondering whether or not it'll be safe to do so."

"Given that you were so often placed in untenable situations by parents who were masters of the double bind, of course you find yourself desperately wanting to avoid that now but assuming that here too you'll eventually find yourself in a no-win situation. The story of your life."

By offering the patient a legitimization statement that validates the way the patient now feels, the therapist is attempting to make it easier for the patient to get in touch with the illusions and distortions that shape his experience of himself and his world. The therapist hopes that the patient, in response to such an intervention, will go on either to elaborate upon the nature of his feelings in the here and now or to recover significant memories from his childhood (and reexperience them).

WHAT IS A MODIFICATION STATEMENT?

The patient's attention is directed inward and backward by way of both distortion statements (that highlight the patient's negative expectations) and legitimization statements (that contextualize these expectations as valid responses to early-on toxic experiences at the hands of the infantile object). Both interventions prompt the patient to observe the fact of his unconscious repetitions; his attention is drawn to the fact that he does rather tend to assume that his objects in the here and now will turn out to be like the bad parent early on, understandable reactions to be sure but of note nonetheless.

In addition to interventions that direct the patient's attention inward and backward, the therapist formulates interventions that focus the patient's attention outward, in order to experience the reality of who the therapist is. A modification statement does just that.

Whereas distortion and legitimization statements avoid addressing the reality of who the therapist actually is (they simply draw the patient's attention to the fact that he does rather tend to have certain expectations about his contemporary objects that would seem to derive from early-on bad experiences), modification statements do focus the patient's attention more directly on the reality of who the therapist is. Modification statements gently challenge the patient's projections by confronting the patient with the reality of who the therapist actually is; more accurately, modification statements confront the patient with *what the patient knows* to be the reality of who the therapist actually is.

A modification statement, therefore, is a particularly useful tool for the working through of negative transference. First it directs the patient's attention outward, to observe the reality of who the therapist actually is; then it resonates with the patient's actual (distorted) experience of the therapist as the bad parent he once had.

Admittedly, the patient responds with distress, fear, upset, or anger when he experiences the therapist as the bad parent he once had. On the other hand, there is something deeply reassuring and nonthreatening about this situation, which is so familiar — even if painful.

Responses that are more positive than what had been expected challenge the patient's characteristic ways of experiencing himself and his objects—in other words, the reality of who the therapist actually is challenges the patient's distortions—and makes him anxious. And so it is that modification statements first name the patient's knowledge of reality (which makes him anxious because of its newness and its challenging of what's tried and true, even if painful) and then name the patient's distorted experience of it (which eases his anxiety by reassuring him with its familiarity).

The format of a prototypical modification statement is as follows:

"Even though you know that . . . , nonetheless your fear is that . . . "

Modification statements first direct the patient's attention to something the patient would rather not be reminded of and then resonate with where the patient is. They strive first to enhance his knowledge (by addressing his observing ego) and then to validate his experience (by addressing his experiencing ego).

Examples of modification statements:

"Although you know that I do not try to control you, you find yourself fearing that I (like your father) might try to tell you what to do."

"Although you know that I have never ridiculed you, you hold back in here for fear that I might think something you were saying was silly or even laughable."

"Even though you know that I am not someone who takes what you say lightly, your fear is that I (like your mother) might not take it seriously."

"Even though you know that I do listen and do understand, at times like this you begin to feel that maybe I don't understand, never have understood, and never will."

"Although you know that I do not sit in judgment, you get worried that I (like your mother) might think ill of you were you to expose how you really feel."

The modification statements above more obviously challenge the patient's distorted perceptions of the therapist (and indirectly, therefore, the patient's misperceptions of himself). By way of example, in the first situation the therapist is challenging the patient's

RESPONDING TO THE PATIENT

unrealistically negative perception of the therapist as like the powerfully controlling father; indirectly, he is also suggesting that the patient's experience of himself as a helpless victim of external forces is also suspect.

Modification statements can also more obviously challenge the patient's distorted perceptions of himself (and indirectly, therefore, the patient's inaccurate perceptions of the therapist). The following modification statements are examples:

"Even though you know that you have a choice about how you use these sessions, you feel sometimes that it is I who have the control."

"Although a part of you is willing to entertain the idea that you may not be quite as helpless as you had thought you were, the rest of you is not yet willing to embrace that idea entirely."

"Even though you know that it's up to you to structure these sessions in a way that will be useful to you, you find yourself looking to me to give you direction and focus."

Modification statements, therefore, challenge (either directly or indirectly) the patient's distorted perceptions of both himself and the therapist.

By way of modification statements, the therapist is attempting to put a wedge between the patient's knowledge of reality (his dawning recognition that the therapist is a new good object) and his negative experience of it (his assumption that the therapist is an old bad object). The therapist is striving to create tension within the patient between his attachment to the present and his loyalty to the past—ultimately, tension within the patient between reality and defense.

IS A MODIFICATION STATEMENT A PARTICULAR KIND OF CONFLICT STATEMENT?

Yes, a modification statement is a particular kind of conflict statement: a conflict statement juxtaposes the patient's knowledge of reality with his experience of it; a modification statement juxtaposes the patient's knowledge of reality with his negative experience of it. Like all other conflict statements, the modification statement first names an anxiety-provoking reality that the patient, on some level, does know and then names the anxiety-assuaging defense (the distortion) to which the patient clings in order not to have to know.

WHAT IS AN INVERTED MODIFICATION STATEMENT?

Early on in the treatment the patient is invested more in his defenses than in reality, tied more to the past than to the present. But with time, by way of statements that direct the patient's attention both inward and backward and by way of statements that direct the patient's attention outward, the patient's attachment to reality becomes more solid and his attachment to his defenses becomes more conflicted. In other words, with time and increased insight, the defense itself begins to provoke some anxiety; as the patient comes to understand both his investment in the defense and the price he pays for maintaining such an investment, the defense becomes increasingly ego-dystonic. No longer does it serve him as it once did.

There comes a time when it provokes more anxiety for the patient to be reminded of his attachment to his defense than for him to be reminded of reality, more anxiety for him to be reminded of how loyal he has been to what's old (and bad) than for him to be reminded of what's new (and good).

At this later point, the patient may be ready for an inverted modification statement, wherein the therapist inverts the order in which he names the two sides of the patient's conflict. Whereas a modification statement addresses first the patient's capacity and then his need, first his healthy capacity to know and then his defensive need not to know, an inverted modification statement first acknowledges the patient's reluctance to let go of his attachment to the past and then resonates with the healthy force within the patient that is in touch with the present, getting ever more powerful, and gaining ever more momentum.

But now it is the patient's pathological attachment to what's old and bad that makes him anxious, his healthy attachment to what's new and good that relieves his anxiety. Now it is the patient's resistance to change that generates anxiety, his wish to change that eases it.

In the pairs that follow, the first is a modification statement and the second an inverted modification statement:

1. "Even though you know that I would not laugh at you, you hold back in here for fear that I might."
2. "Sometimes you hold back in here for fear that I might laugh at you, but you are coming to know that I would not really do that."

1. "Although you are beginning to realize that I may be more trustworthy than you had originally thought, at this point you are not yet sure that I am really someone whom you will be able to trust."
2. "You are not yet sure that I am really someone whom you will be able to trust, but you are beginning to realize that I may be more trustworthy than you had originally thought."

Both of these inverted modification statements are addressed to a patient who is becoming more and more able to acknowledge the reality of who the therapist actually is, uncontaminated by his need for the therapist to be otherwise. Now it makes the patient more anxious to be reminded of his investment in his fear than to be reminded of reality. At this point, the patient has already begun to change, to let go of his investment in the past, to relinquish his attachment to the infantile object, to overcome his resistance, and to move forward in the treatment and in his life.

WHAT IS A FACILITATION STATEMENT?

More generally, the patient's forward movement in the treatment and in his life is fostered by way of facilitation statements, in which the therapist articulates both the patient's healthy wish to feel or to do something and the unhealthy fears that interfere with his feeling or doing that something; in a facilitation statement, then, the therapist makes explicit both the patient's desire and his fear.

The therapist wants, ultimately, to broaden and deepen the patient's understanding of his internal psychodynamics, both the healthy wishes that motivate him and the unhealthy fears that interfere with the actualization of such wishes.

By way of facilitation statements, the therapist is attempting to facilitate ultimate resolution of the patient's underlying conflict by juxtaposing the patient's healthy wish to change with his unhealthy fears about changing. The therapist wants the patient to recognize that he is motivated by healthy forces but that he resists forward movement because he is frightened.

Part of what fuels the patient's unhealthy fear may be the distorted perceptions he has of himself and his own abilities. He may be unable to move forward in his life because he is held back by negative misperceptions about himself, distortions that arise from having taken upon himself the burden of his parent's limitations, distortions that now fuel his sense of himself as inadequate and, therefore, his reluctance to go for it.

In a facilitation statement, the therapist is hoping to facilitate exploration of such defenses, so that they can ultimately be worked through and overcome and so that the patient's healthy wish to realize his potential can rise to the fore.

Examples of facilitation statements:

"You would like to be able to trust me, but you are afraid that you may never be able to forgive me for what I did."

"You would like to be able to move beyond how upset you are with me, but you are very angry and cannot imagine that you will ever be able to work through your disappointment."

"You would like to be able to believe in this process, but you are afraid to let yourself have hope."

"You would like to be able to commit to coming regularly to our sessions, but you hold back for fear that you'll be disappointed."

"You would like to be able to share parts of yourself that you usually keep hidden, but you get anxious when you think about doing that."

There are, of course, unhealthy, neurotic, infantile wishes that motivate patients (and that they are conflicted about); in a facilitation statement, however, the focus (in the first part) is upon the healthy, growth-promoting wishes that motivate the patient to actualize his potential.

RESPONDING TO THE PATIENT

By the same token, there are, of course, healthy fears that interfere with the patient's realization of his potential; in a facilitation statement, however, the emphasis (in the second part) is upon the unhealthy, neurotic, infantile fears (distortions) that need eventually to be explored and relinquished before the patient's resistance to moving in the direction of health can be overcome.

By way of a facilitation statement, the therapist is giving the patient permission to expound upon either his healthy wish to change or his unhealthy resistance to change.

IS A FACILITATION STATEMENT A PARTICULAR KIND OF CONFLICT STATEMENT?

A facilitation statement resembles a conflict statement in that (1) it concerns itself with explicating both sides of the patient's conflict about moving forward in the treatment and in his life and (2) it names first the healthy, growth-promoting "Yes" force (that constitutes the patient's mental health) and then the unhealthy, growth-inhibiting "No" force (that constitutes the patient's pathology or resistance).

In important ways, then, a facilitation statement has the same format as a conflict statement. There are, however, a few interesting differences, perhaps mostly in emphasis.

Whereas the first part of a conflict statement usually names what the patient would really rather the therapist not name, the first part of a facilitation statement names a healthy wish that the patient may have much less trouble acknowledging the presence of.

Whereas the first part of a conflict statement articulates a force that provokes anxiety and therefore needs to be defended against, the first part of a facilitation statement names a motivating force that provokes much less anxiety and, therefore, much less a need for defense.

Whereas a conflict statement first challenges a defense and then supports it, a facilitation statement is less intent upon creating such tension. A facilitation statement strives simply to get named both the "Yes" force that motivates movement toward health and the "No" force that resists such movement. The "No" may arise in response to the presence of the "Yes" force (in which case we are dealing with convergent conflict) or it may exist independently of the "Yes" force (in which case we are dealing with divergent conflict).

Finally, a conflict statement highlights the tension between what the patient knows (even if sometimes he would rather forget) and what the patient feels, in order to make the patient's experience increasingly anxiety-provoking; a facilitation statement, however, is designed not so much to create further conflict as to explicate both sides of the conflict that already exists between healthy wish and unhealthy fear, between desire for change and resistance to it.

Perhaps, then, we could think of facilitation statements as constituting a subclass of conflict statements. Both interventions name the two sides of the patient's conflict about overcoming his resistance and moving toward health; but the facilitation statement does so more with an eye to facilitating the patient's recognition of both his desire to get better and his fears about getting better, whereas the conflict statement attempts to create tension within the patient between his knowledge of reality and his experience of it.

III

Clinical Practice

NINE

The Cocoon Transference

IS THE TRANSFERENCE AN ASPECT OF THE RESISTANCE?

In previous chapters, we have suggested that the transference, more specifically, the transferential need to experience one's objects as either the good parent one did not have or the bad parent one did have, fuels the resistance.

But, as with all aspects of the resistance, the transference (whether positive or negative) is double-edged. On the one hand, the transference obstructs the patient's forward movement in the treatment and in his life by interfering with the patient's capacity to experience his objects as they really are. On the other hand, the transference creates opportunity where before there was none — because it is the working through of the transference that is the process by which new good structure is added (structural growth) and old bad structure is altered (structural change).

Furthermore, whereas the patient in the early stages of the treatment may resist mobilization of the transference, at a later stage in the treatment the patient may well resist its resolution. In other words, the patient may initially be reluctant to deliver himself into the transference but later become so entrenched in it that he finds himself reluctant to get out.

In fact, the hallmark of a patient in the throes of a positive transference is the intensity with which he clings to his infantile wishes and the relentlessness with which he pursues their gratification by the therapist. The hallmark of a patient in the throes of a negative transference is the intensity with which he clings to his infantile fears and the compulsive repetitiveness with which he recapitulates, in the treatment situation, his unresolved childhood dramas. Such patients cannot confront the reality of who their objects are—whether the infantile object or, now, the transference object; they experience reality as they need it to be.

But no real structural work can be accomplished unless the patient can tolerate first having the need (whether for good or for bad) and then giving it up.

WITH WHAT KIND OF POWER DOES THE PATIENT VEST THE THERAPIST?

Part of what enables the therapist to be effective (whether in his capacity as the good parent the patient never had or the bad parent the patient did have) is that he comes to assume the importance of the original parent. When the therapist has been vested with such power, then and only then is the patient's relationship with the therapist able to serve as a corrective for damage sustained early on at the hands of the parent. And it is by way of internalizing aspects of this new relationship that the patient's internal world can be modified and the patient healed.

Interestingly, because the parent in the here and now is no longer imbued with the same power he was once imbued with, now the parent has much less power to heal than once the parent had power to hurt. It is therefore not so much the contemporary parent who can make the difference in the patient's life as it is the therapist, who operates in the place of the original parent. It is because the therapist comes to assume the significance of the original parent that the therapist has both the power to heal and the power to harm.

WHY DO PATIENTS RESIST DELIVERING THEMSELVES AND THEIR VULNERABILITIES INTO THE TREATMENT SITUATION?

For the therapist to be able to make a real difference (in terms of the structural configuration of the patient's internal world), the therapist must have come to assume the importance of the infantile object.

But the patient may resist having such a close relationship with his therapist; he may be unable to tolerate the anxiety attendant upon making himself that vulnerable. The patient's concern may be with losing control, regressing, or becoming too dependent. The patient may be profoundly fearful that, were he to deliver himself and his needs into the relationship, he would expose himself to the possibility of further traumatic disappointment, injury, and heartache—and the thought of that is intolerable.

WHAT IS THE DEFENSE OF AFFECTIVE NONRELATEDNESS?

To describe such a state of affairs, Arnold Modell (1975) has suggested use of the term *cocoon transference*. The patient clings to illusions of grandiose self-sufficiency; he would like to believe that he needs no one and that he can be the source of his own emotional sustenance. The struggle is to maintain his precariously established sense of autonomy and the fear is that expressing intense affect will lead to dissolution of the integrity and cohesiveness of the self.

Modell describes the patient's stance in the opening phase of the treatment as a narcissistic defense against affects, a state of affective nonrelatedness. The patient himself often reports feeling that he is encased in a "plastic bubble" or a "bell jar"; and, at later stages in the treatment, whenever the patient is narcissistically injured, he withdraws into his cocoon, retreats into his splendid isolation, denies any need for the therapist.

In fact, the patient's transferential need for the therapist to be both the good parent he never had and the bad parent he did have may be present from the very start. But, as long as the patient resists affective engagement with the therapist, he will be reluctant to acknowledge the existence of such needs.

HOW IS THE PATIENT CONFLICTED IN THE INITIAL STAGES OF THE TREATMENT?

There are many patients, then, for whom the conflict, at least initially, is around having any kind of real relationship with the therapist. Although on some level the patient yearns to be close, on another level the patient is terrified of being close. In other words, the healthy forces within the patient press for intimacy and connection, but the unhealthy forces defend against such longings and resist such connection.

HOW DOES THE THERAPIST RESPOND TO THE PATIENT'S DENIAL OF OBJECT NEED?

In the interest of highlighting those defenses that the therapist senses are interfering with the patient's delivery of himself and his vulnerabilities into the treatment situation, the therapist may say any of the following:

"You are not sure that you want to be in the position of needing me."

"You are determined not to let me matter that much."

"It's hard to think about needing anyone."

"You are reluctant to be in the position of needing anybody right now."

"You are not convinced that it is yet safe enough to have those kinds of feelings in here with me."

"You do not want to be missing me while I'm away this summer."

Each of these statements is an instance of going with the resistance; the resistance is being named, in an experience-near, nonshaming fashion. The patient's defensive need to avoid genuine contact is supported, reinforced, not challenged. By naming the defense, the therapist is highlighting the fact of it; but by doing it nonjudgmentally, the therapist is giving the patient permission to have such a need, without having to justify it.

> **HOW DOES THE THERAPIST CONVEY HIS APPRECIATION FOR HOW INVESTED THE PATIENT MAY BE IN HIS DEFENSES?**

The therapist may choose to do more than simply name the fact of the defense; he may want to say things that indicate to the patient just how much he appreciates the patient's investment in maintaining his autonomy, remaining in control, and needing no one, least of all the therapist.

"You pride yourself on your ability to be self-sufficient, to do it by yourself."

"You enjoy the feeling of being on your own and are not about to give that up."

"You have worked hard to create a life for yourself in which you do not really have to depend upon anyone."

It is important that the patient, eventually, come to understand more about the unhealthy resistive forces that interfere with the delivery of himself and his needs into the relationship with the therapist. And if the legitimacy of the defense is not challenged, the patient may be able to elaborate upon his need for the defense. He may associate to why he has come to need the defense and how it now serves him.

HOW ARE FACILITATION STATEMENTS USEFUL?

The therapist may also want to use a facilitation statement, in which he articulates the patient's internal dilemma about allowing himself to be close, known, understood, held. It is important that the therapist make explicit both sides of the conflict the patient is struggling with — both his desire for closeness and his fear of closeness.

So the therapist, in the interest of facilitating the patient's delivery of himself into the relationship, makes statements that highlight first the patient's wish to be close and then his fears about being close:

> "There may be times when you find yourself yearning to be known and understood; but, for the most part, you can't imagine ever being able to let someone get that close."
>
> "A part of you wants so much to be able to trust me, but another part of you is scared and is not at all sure that you want ever again to be in the position of depending upon anybody."
>
> "You want desperately to be understood, but you also find yourself wanting to remain hidden, not exposed, not vulnerable. Alone, but safe."
>
> "You would wish that you could count on somebody else for a change, but you have managed thus far on your own and you're not sure you feel comfortable changing that now."
>
> "Perhaps you would want to be able to open yourself up to the possibility of a relationship, but it feels safer somehow to remain cautious and to proceed at your own pace."

In general, as Modell (1975) so poignantly observes, the therapist must use his intuition to assess whether, at any given moment in time, the patient needs to be found or needs to remain unfound, not known.

HOW ARE LEGITIMIZATION STATEMENTS USEFUL?

Legitimization statements can be used in conjunction with facilitation statements to encourage the patient's delivery of himself into the

THE COCOON TRANSFERENCE

treatment situation. They attempt to put into historical perspective both the patient's yearnings to be close and his fears about such closeness.

In the following statements, the patient's longing is contextualized as an understandable response to early-on injury:

"Given that you felt so misunderstood by your mother, of course you long to be able to find that understanding now."

"Because you were so hurt by your father whom you loved so, of course you find yourself wanting to make sure that you'll be safe in here with me."

In the following statements, the patient's fear is contextualized as a legitimate response to early-on disappointment:

"Given that you felt so misunderstood by your mother, of course your fear is that I too will let you down in that way."

"Because you were so hurt by your father whom you adored, of course you are fearful that you will be hurt by me as well."

Or, the therapist may offer the patient a statement that both legitimizes and facilitates:

"Because you had no one you could depend upon as you were growing up, of course you find yourself wanting desperately now to be able to depend upon me but wondering whether or not it'll be safe to do so."

This statement legitimizes both the patient's hope that maybe this time it will be different and his fear that perhaps it won't.

HOW ARE WORK-TO-BE-DONE CONFLICT STATEMENTS USEFUL?

The therapist may make statements in which he first directs the patient's attention to where the therapist wants the patient to be and then resonates with where the patient is:

"You know that eventually, to overcome your fears of intimacy, you will have to let someone in, but right now you're feeling that you simply cannot afford to take the risk of being hurt again."

"You know that eventually you're going to have to let me in, but right now you're not yet ready to take the chance."

"You know that you may someday need to let this relationship be important to you, but you are hoping that you'll be able to get the work done without ever having to let me matter all that much."

Such statements first spell out the work the patient must eventually do to overcome his fears of intimacy and then acknowledge the fact of the patient's fears.

HOW IS THE PATIENT'S AFFECTIVE NONENGAGEMENT FINALLY WORKED THROUGH?

The patient is being given permission to remember old injuries, old disappointments, old pain. It is important that he be able to feel, in the here and now, some of the upset, anguish, and rage he felt as a child in relation to his traumatically disappointing parents.

And, as he begins to understand the origins of his need to have others not matter — namely, that it is too scary to let them in — his need to maintain his distance diminishes and the defense of affective nonrelatedness becomes less necessary.

As the defense becomes less necessary, the patient becomes more ready to look at the ways in which the therapist has come to matter to him — as both the good parent he didn't have and the bad parent he did have.

TEN

The Positive Transference and Its Disruptions

In a recent *New Yorker* cartoon, a gentleman, seated at a table in a restaurant by the name of The Disillusionment Cafe, is awaiting the arrival of his order. His waiter returns to his table and announces, "Your order is not ready, nor will it ever be."

HOW DOES THE POSITIVE TRANSFERENCE EMERGE?

As we discussed earlier, with respect to drive theory, positive transference is thought to result from the patient's delivery (by way of displacement) of his libidinal and aggressive needs into the relationship with the therapist. Where once the parent was the drive object, now the therapist becomes the drive object; as such, the therapist is experienced either as actually gratifying the patient's need (in the present) or as potentially gratifying (at some point in the future). In the literature, such a transference is usually described as a neurotic transference.

With respect to self theory, positive transference is thought to result from the patient's delivery (by way of displacement) of his narcissistic needs into the relationship with the therapist. Where once the parent was the selfobject, now the therapist becomes the selfobject; as such, the therapist is experienced either as actually gratifying the patient's need for perfection (in the present) or as potentially gratifying (at some point in the future). In the literature, such a transference is usually described as a selfobject (or narcissistic) transference.

Because self theory spells out so nicely the relationship between working through, or grieving, the loss of transference illusions (optimal disillusionment) and the laying down of new good structure (transmuting internalization), we now examine in some detail the process by which disruptions of the selfobject transference are worked through and structural growth is effected. This working-through process informs our understanding, more generally, of the process by which infantile needs (be they narcissistic or libidinal/aggressive) are transformed into mature capacity (be it in the form of self structure or drive structure).

WHAT HAPPENS TO FRUSTRATED NEED?

To review, when there is the experience of nontraumatic frustration of infantile need (frustration that can be worked through and mastered), then there is both impetus and opportunity for the adding of new good structure (be it self structure or drive structure) by way of transforming the need. In other words, nontraumatically frustrated needs are gradually tamed, modified, and integrated as healthy structure (capacity).

When, however, there is the experience of traumatic frustration of infantile need (frustration that cannot be worked through and mastered), then there is no such impetus, no such opportunity, and no such transformation of energy into structure, need into capacity. Not only is there no taming of the need but it is reinforced. We had earlier suggested that traumatically thwarted psychological (develop mental) needs become narcissistic needs and traumatically thwarted physiological (libidinal/aggressive) needs become neurotic needs.

WHAT IS BENEVOLENT CONTAINMENT?

With respect to psychological needs, *optimal disillusionment* is the term used by the self psychologists to describe nontraumatic frustration (whether by the selfobject parent of the child's developmental needs or by the selfobject therapist of the patient's narcissistic needs). With respect to physiological needs, the term I would like to propose to describe nontraumatic frustration (whether by the infantile drive object of the child's libidinal/aggressive needs or by the drive object therapist of the patient's neurotic needs) is *benevolent containment.*

In other words, I am suggesting that we think of optimal disillusionment of psychological needs and benevolent containment of physiological needs as the heroes in this piece. And whether we are speaking of disillusionment that is optimal or containment that is benevolent, it is the fact of the frustration and its eventual working through that is the process by which need is transformed into capacity, energy into structure.

WHAT IS AN IMPORTANT DIFFERENCE BETWEEN PSYCHOLOGICAL AND PHYSIOLOGICAL NEEDS?

There is, however, a crucial distinction to be made between psychological needs and physiological needs. Whereas the parent's responsibility is to do what he can to gratify the child's developmental needs and the therapist's responsibility is to do what he can to gratify the patient's narcissistic needs, it is the parent's responsibility, ultimately, to frustrate the child's libidinal/aggressive needs and the therapist's responsibility, ultimately, to frustrate the patient's neurotic needs.

In other words, the working-through process (with respect to both the psychological needs of self theory and the physiological needs of drive theory) involves frustration against a backdrop of gratification. But, whereas the selfobject should do the best he can to gratify the psychological needs (the frustration of them will be inevitable), the drive object must appreciate that, sooner rather than later, the physiological needs must be frustrated. It is then the working through of such frustration (whether of the psychological needs or the physiological needs) that is the occasion for structural growth.

In summary, whereas the psychological needs must be gratified, the physiological needs must be frustrated.

WHAT ARE ID NEEDS AND WHAT ARE EGO NEEDS?

Along similar lines, Winnicott has suggested that we think of the patient as having different kinds of needs: id needs (which relate to instinctual gratification) and ego needs (which relate to the need for objects, the need for connection with—and recognition by—objects). The id needs are physiological and the ego needs are more psychological.

If an id need is frustrated, the patient experiences rage. The rage experienced by the patient in the here and now belongs in part to the current frustrating situation but in larger part to the original traumatic failure situation. Winnicott (1963a) says there is thus an opportunity for the patient to rework the original trauma by working through rage experienced in relation to the therapist.

Whereas id needs can be frustrated, ego needs must never be frustrated. If an ego need is not met, the result is not rage but retraumatization, a reinforcement of the original traumatic failure situation.

WHY DO WE TURN TO SELF PSYCHOLOGY?

Whether the need is physiological or psychological, neurotic or narcissistic, id or ego, whether the need must be initially frustrated or initially gratified and then frustrated, it is the process of working through that frustration that enables the person to separate and grow. Again, because self theory explicates so beautifully the details of this working-through process, we will rely upon what it has to say about that process to help us understand how the patient's needs are tamed and integrated as psychic structure. We will see how such a transformation enables the patient to renounce his need for infantile gratification, to relinquish his ties to the past, to develop the capacity to be more fully present in the here and now, and to free himself up to move forward toward the realization of his potential—in other words, to overcome his resistance.

The process of transformation is a grieving process, a process of gradual disillusionment. Confronting the reality of who the patient's objects are (both past and present) and experiencing the pain of his disappointment are at the heart of the healing process. Development of capacity is the result.

In what follows, then, we will explore the working-through process from the self psychological perspective of the patient with structural deficit (impaired capacity) who, in order to compensate for underlying feelings of worthlessness and inadequacy, is relentless in his pursuit of perfection, within both himself and his objects.

Self psychology speaks usually to the patient's narcissistic need for perfection; sometimes, however, it speaks more generally to the patient's narcissistic need for external reinforcement (or regulation) of his self-esteem—or his narcissistic need for empathic recognition. Strictly speaking, then, the patient's need is for perfection and his impaired capacity relates to his inability to tolerate imperfection; loosely speaking, the patient's need is for external regulation of his self-esteem and his impaired capacity relates to his inability to provide such regulation internally. The context usually makes clear the nature of the need.

HOW DOES A NARCISSISTIC PATIENT WITH STRUCTURAL DEFICIT INITIALLY PRESENT?

When a patient has structural deficit, he has trouble feeling good about himself. When such a patient presents to treatment, typically his chief complaints reflect his internal sense of vulnerability and impoverishment; he generally reports overwhelming feelings of hopelessness, helplessness, and despair. He is often either profoundly anxious or profoundly depressed.

He generally lacks vitality, a feeling of aliveness; he may describe himself as feeling wooden or dead inside. He gets little pleasure or sense of prideful accomplishment from his life; he is chronically dissatisfied and unhappy.

HOW DOES THE PATIENT'S NEED FOR PERFECTION MANIFEST ITSELF IN THE TRANSFERENCE?

Once there has been resolution of the patient's reluctance to deliver himself, his affect, and his vulnerabilities into the treatment situation, the patient's archaic narcissistic needs (his thwarted developmental needs that had long ago been split off and repressed) become reactivated in the therapeutic situation. The therapist now gains access to what would otherwise remain a closed system.

When the patient uses the therapist as a selfobject (as a narcissistic extension of himself), we speak of a selfobject (or narcissistic) transference. The therapist is experienced as the embodiment of a particular psychological function that the patient is lacking. He is used to provide narcissistic gratification—enhancement of the patient's sense of perfection (strictly speaking) or enhancement of the patient's self-esteem (loosely speaking). More specifically, a selfobject is used to provide self-regulation because such regulation cannot be provided internally. Selfobjects fill in for missing psychic structure (missing capacity); in essence, they function as precursors of psychic structure.

We speak of a mirror transference when the grandiose self becomes therapeutically remobilized. The grandiose self insists upon mirroring confirmation of its perfection by the mirroring selfobject.

We speak of an idealizing transference when the idealized selfobject becomes therapeutically reactivated. The function performed by the idealized selfobject therapist is provision of an opportunity for the patient to invest his objects with perfection, so that he can look up to them as a source of inspiration, guidance, strength, and power.

WHAT DO WE MEAN BY A SECOND CHANCE?

Through the relationship with the selfobject therapist, there is an opportunity for the patient with structural deficit (or developmental arrest) to continue the growth process interrupted years earlier because of traumatic disenchantment with the parents. There is a developmental opportunity for a new beginning, a filling in, firming, and consolidation of the self, a repair or restoration of the injured, damaged self — by way of internalizing aspects of the relationship with the selfobject therapist. Internalized functions become psychic structures; in this way, the erstwhile external goodness is internally recorded and preserved.

WHAT IS THE ROLE OF ILLUSION IN A NARCISSISTIC TRANSFERENCE?

The patient's experience of the therapist is either "You, the therapist, are the perfect parent I never had" or "My hope is that you will someday become the perfect parent I never had." In either situation, the object is experienced, in an unrealistically positive way, as the good/perfect parent the patient never had.

Illusion is ultimately involved in such transferences. Although it may seem that the patient is looking to the therapist for something that is entirely reasonable (like understanding, reassurance, help), in fact it will usually be found that the patient is looking to the therapist to be the perfect parent he never had and to make up for the early-on bad parenting. It is this fantasy that is unrealistic, this hope that is illusory. In fact, the therapist may share the patient's fantasy; the therapist may also believe that he (the therapist) can, and should, make up the difference to the patient.

But, although both patient and therapist might wish it to be that way, it doesn't work like that. And it will be as the patient confronts the reality of his disenchantment that structural growth will occur and his need for illusion will become transformed into a capacity to experience reality as it is. It will be as the patient works through his disillusionment that he will overcome his resistance and get better.

WHAT IF THE THERAPIST'S FAILURES ARE TRAUMATIC ONES?

In this book, our focus is upon those failures by the therapist that the patient can ultimately work through and master—namely, nontraumatic or optimal disillusionments. When the therapist, for whatever the reason, fails the patient in traumatic ways, we are no longer simply talking about a situation of transference (in which the assumption is that the patient's perceptions of the therapist are unrealistic and inappropriate). When the therapist participates in ways that the patient cannot process and master, then the situation is much more complicated and one that is well beyond the scope of this primer.

HOW IS THE ILLUSION STATEMENT USEFUL?

When the patient's archaic narcissistic needs have been therapeutically remobilized and delivered into the treatment situation, the patient is in a vulnerable position in relation to the therapist. The therapist must be ever respectful of that. By way of illusion statements that name, but do not challenge, the patient's magical expectations with respect to the therapist, the therapist is able to resonate empathically with where the patient is and what the patient's experience is of the therapist.

Examples of illusion statements:

"You are enjoying the feeling that you are in safe hands and will not be hurt here."

"You are hoping that I will be able to offer you interpretations that will enable you to gain more access to your past."

"You want me to give you insight."

"You are hoping that this therapy will be very different from the other ones."

"You are hoping that I will know where to go from here."

"You are hoping that I will be able to say things to help you get more in touch with how you're feeling."

"You had never thought that you would ever again be able to feel this hopeful."

"When you're feeling this good, you can't imagine that I could ever let you down."

When the therapist is understanding that the patient's positive feelings about the therapist as the good parent he didn't have are beginning to wane, illusion statements are also facilitative. To facilitate the eventual working through of the disrupted positive transference, the therapist may intervene as follows:

"You were so hoping that I would not fail you as the others before me had failed you."

"You had so hoped that I would not make the same kinds of mistakes that everybody else had made."

"You were feeling hopeful for the first time in years."

"You were delighted that you had finally found someone by whom you could feel accepted."

"It had felt so good to be knowing that you were understood."

WHAT IS THE ROLE OF ENTITLEMENT IN A NARCISSISTIC TRANSFERENCE?

Sometimes a patient, in the throes of a narcissistic transference, becomes quite entitled, expectant, demanding, insistent, relentless. Because the internal experience of structural deficit is that there are gaps, holes, an inner void, an absence of internal resources, the patient may become quite explicit that he wants the therapist to give him things that will enable him to feel more complete. He wants the difference made up to him and demands that the therapist be the one to do it.

And so the patient asks that the therapist do this, that he do that. The patient may demand reassurance, answers, guarantees. The patient may insist that he be held, that he be told he is special, that he be told he is loved. The patient is not trying to be difficult; the patient simply cannot do these things on his own—and so looks to the outside for the provision of what he himself lacks. The patient's refrain may go something like this: "I want this, I need that, I demand that you give me this, I insist that you offer me that." The patient wants gratification of his infantile needs; he expects such gratification, and he feels entitled to get it now.

HOW IS THE ENTITLEMENT STATEMENT USEFUL?

In the face of the patient's entitled sense that he is owed all sorts of things by the therapist to compensate for early-on privation, deprivation, and injury, the therapist may use entitlement statements, in which he names, nonjudgmentally, the fact of the patient's entitlement. The therapist is acknowledging not only that the patient hopes the therapist will be able to make up the difference to him but that the patient feels entitled to such compensation because he felt so cheated as a child.

Examples of entitlement statements:

"You are feeling that I should be able to understand without having to hear further details."

"You are feeling that it is my responsibility to ask you questions."

"You feel that I owe it to you to answer all your questions directly."

"You believe that I ought to be able to say things that will make you feel better."

"You are thinking that it is not unreasonable to be expecting that, at this point, I be willing to offer you some reassurance about your prognosis."

"You are feeling that I should be helping you to remember more details about the abuse."

"You feel that I should know when to ask you questions and when to be silent."

WHAT IS THE DEFENSE OF RELENTLESS ENTITLEMENT?

A patient in the throes of a narcissistic transference may get caught up in something I refer to as relentless entitlement, more specifically, the defense of relentless entitlement. The patient employs this defense to protect himself against the experience of frustration; the patient cannot confront the pain of being disappointed—and so defends himself against such pain by clinging to his relentless entitlement, his refusal to take "No" for an answer.

When the patient delivers his relentless entitlement into the treatment situation, the patient becomes deeply convinced that the therapist could gratify a particular need—but chooses not to, that the therapist has the capacity to give the patient something he desperately wants—but refuses to. The patient feels entitled to have his need met; he is relentless in his pursuit of it and outraged in the face of its being denied.

This stalemated situation (and the sadomasochistic dynamics that often underlie it) requires a more aggressive approach than is ordinarily required in working through the patient's defensive need for illusion.

HOW IS THE LEGITIMIZATION STATEMENT USEFUL?

In addition to illusion and entitlement statements, legitimization statements can be used to validate the patient's wishes and magical expectations with respect to the therapist. The therapist, by framing the patient's illusions and entitlement as an understandable reaction to early-on traumatically heartbreaking experiences, is able both to enhance the patient's knowledge of himself and to validate the patient's experience.

Examples of legitimization statements:

"Given that you never really felt known and understood as a child, of course you find yourself desperately wanting that from me now."

"Because your parents gave you so little recognition when you were young, of course you find yourself craving that attention and recognition now."

"Given that you were never able to feel safe as a young child, of course you find yourself wishing that you could feel that now."

"Given that when you were young you were never made to feel special, of course now you yearn to be told that are special."

"Given that you were never able to know if your parents were proud of you, of course you find yourself feeling the need for such reassurance from me now."

"Because you never knew whether or not your mother really loved you, of course now you find yourself feeling that you cannot know for sure that I love you unless I tell you that I do."

By way of illusion statements, entitlement statements, and legitimization statements, the therapist is striving to make the patient ever more aware of the ways in which he is always yearning for his objects to be other than, better than, more perfect than, they really are.

HOW DO ILLUSION, ENTITLEMENT, AND LEGITIMIZATION STATEMENTS LAY THE GROUNDWORK FOR THE EVENTUAL WORKING THROUGH OF THE PATIENT'S DISILLUSIONMENT?

By way of illusion, entitlement, and legitimization statements, the therapist is highlighting the fact of the patient's expectations with respect to the therapy and the therapist — expectations that are magical, as it happens, but that is not the main thrust of these interventions. The therapist is striving to increase the patient's level of awareness about the illusions to which he clings, whether the illusions relate to the infantile object, the transference object, or a contemporary object.

The therapist wants to encourage the patient to elaborate upon the illusions around which he has unconsciously organized his experience of the world and to make the patient more aware of the longings he brings to the therapy and to his relationship with the therapist.

Acknowledgment of (illusory) hope is important foundation work for the patient's working through of his eventual, and inevitable, disillusionment, when it turns out that the therapist is not as good (perfect) as the patient would have hoped. It is, of course, by way of working through such disappointments, by way of working through such disruptions of the positive transference, that the patient will be able, in time, to give up his illusions and overcome this aspect of his resistance.

HOW DOES THE PATIENT RESPOND TO INTERVENTIONS THAT DIRECT HIS ATTENTION AWAY FROM WHERE HE IS IN THE MOMENT?

When the patient delivers his need for the good (perfect) parent he never had into the transference and basks in the warm glow of feeling that he has finally found what he has been searching for all his life, then it is important that the therapist make a very real effort to be with the patient where he is.

If the therapist attempts to direct the patient's attention away from where he is in the moment, then such interventions may well be experienced by the patient as intrusive and injurious. The patient would like to be able to feel that he controls everything; therefore, he is threatened when the therapist's comments suggest that the therapist knows something the patient may not yet be aware of. The patient is particularly uncomfortable when genetic interpretations are made about the impact of his past on his present, because such interventions remind him of things that he has little or no control over.

WHAT HAPPENS WHEN THE THERAPIST SERMONIZES?

The therapist must appreciate that, given the patient's underlying feelings of defectiveness and inferiority and given his impaired capacity to be internally self-reinforcing, the patient's need for external reinforcement is entirely understandable, reasonable, and expectable.

Therapists who are not well-versed in self psychology may respond to the narcissistically entitled patient by sermonizing or by urging the patient to moderate his overt displays of contemptuous superiority and haughty arrogance. In essence, the patient is told that his demands are unrealistic and inappropriate; he is shamed into keeping hidden his grandiose claims and infantile expectations.

If the patient complies, then he will no longer appear narcissistic and entitled. But there will have been no real structural work done, and the opportunity will have been lost to transform his entitlement into healthy capacity.

WHAT DOES IT MEAN TO COMPLY WITH THE PATIENT'S NARCISSISTIC DEMANDS?

Rather than confrontation and vigorous interpretation of the patient's narcissistic needs, the therapist allows the need to be. The therapist does not challenge the patient's need for perfection; instead, he does what he can to convey to the patient his respect for the patient's need. Nor does the therapist challenge the patient's need for external reinforcement; instead, he does what he can to resonate empathically with the patient's need to be narcissistically reinforced. By way of illusion, entitlement, and legitimization statements, the therapist supports—and does not confront—the patient's wish for magical fulfillment.

But there may be times when, intuitively, the therapist senses that not only must he understand the patient's need to have his narcissism gratified but also he must actually gratify the patient's narcissism. As an example, the patient who clamors to have the therapist tell him that he is okay even if he has sex with prostitutes may simply need to hear that the therapist thinks he is okay. In other words, sometimes it is sufficient to name the patient's wish to be reassured, but sometimes it is necessary to provide the actual reassurance.

The self psychologists suggest that (reluctant) compliance with the patient's narcissistic need for external reinforcement may sometimes be necessary if the therapist is to avoid retraumatizing the patient.

HOW IS GRATIFICATION OF NEED NECESSARY BUT NOT SUFFICIENT FOR GROWTH?

The self psychologists, for the most part, do not claim that such compliance, on its own, effects actual structural growth. In fact, as we know, the self psychologists believe that gratification is necessary for such growth—but not sufficient; it is frustration against a backdrop of gratification that prompts internalization, the building up of internal structure, the filling in of deficit, and the giving up of infantile need.

WHY DO WE NOT INTERPRET A POSITIVE TRANSFERENCE?

When a narcissistic transference is in place, the patient feels good. At this point it is unnecessary to do any interpreting of the transference—because the patient should be given the opportunity to feel narcissistically gratified and psychologically complete, without being stripped of whatever illusions may be fueling his good feelings.

This is a very different situation indeed from the situation that arises when there is a negative transference, in which the patient re-creates in the here and now the early-on traumatic failure situation. As long as such a transference goes unchallenged, then the patient will be further traumatized.

Whereas negative transferences must therefore be interpreted, positive transferences need not. The patient should be allowed to have the experience of having his needs met (or of having the illusion that his needs will someday be met) so that he will be able to tolerate the inevitable disenchantment, when it turns out that his therapist will not be able to provide for him in all the ways that he would have wanted.

WHY DO WE INTERPRET DISRUPTED POSITIVE TRANSFERENCES?

Only in the context of the therapist's disappointment of the patient is there need for interpretation — to help the patient master his experience of having been failed.

Furthermore, only in the context of the therapist's disappointment of the patient is there the reminder that the object is separate from the self. Whereas gratification fosters good feelings in the patient and provides him with the experience of being understood, validated, and held, frustration brings the patient up short, mobilizes his outrage, and ultimately promotes separation, individuation, and autonomy. Gratification reinforces his feelings of being "at one"; frustration reminds him that this is not so.

WHAT IS THE RELATIONSHIP BETWEEN RECOGNITION OF SEPARATENESS AND CAPACITY TO INTERNALIZE?

Kohut and Winnicott have very different things to say about the relationship between the recognition of separateness and the capacity to internalize. Whereas Kohut believes that internalization precedes separation, Winnicott believes the opposite — that separation precedes internalization.

Kohut suggests that the selfobject is experienced as a part of the self. Optimal disillusionment with the selfobject leads to transmuting internalization, the accretion of internal structure, the filling in of deficit. As this happens, there is no longer the same need to use the object as a selfobject, no longer the same need for a selfobject to complete the self. The object can now be related to in a different way, a way that recognizes the object as separate from the self. Internalization results, therefore, in a capacity to tolerate the separateness between self and object.

But, in marked contrast to this, Winnicott suggests that there is no impetus for internalization until the object is experienced as separate from the self.

Winnicott (1960, 1963a) posited a developmental progression from a stage of absolute dependence (characterized by object relating, in which the mother is experienced as a subjective object indistinguishable from the self), through a stage of relative dependence (characterized by the mother's graduated failure of adaptation, which establishes the fact of her externality), to a stage of autonomy (characterized by object usage, in which the mother can be objectively perceived, is experienced as separate from the self, and is therefore capable of being "used," that is, internalized).

According to Winnicott, then, it is only with achievement of the capacity to recognize mother's separateness that she can be used, or internalized. Winnicott is saying, therefore, that recognition of separateness between self and object precedes internalization.

I had misread Winnicott for years. I had assumed that when he spoke about the holding environment, he was suggesting that the infant is nourished by an environment that provides all sorts of nutrients that can then be absorbed and taken in, as by osmosis.

But Winnicott is not talking about internalization. The maternal holding environment provides a protective envelope within which the so-called inherited potential of the infant can be actualized. The mother does not provide nourishment; she provides protection from impingement. The mother allows her infant the experience of an uninterrupted continuity of being; and, in essence, she facilitates the coming into being of the infant's true self. At this stage of development, internalization is not involved.

It is only later, after the third and final stage of development has been achieved (in which self and object are recognized as separate), that the child can internalize the object. Only when objects have come to be recognized as outside his sphere of omnipotence, as separate from him, does the child develop the capacity to internalize objects.

Achievement of the capacity to recognize the separateness between self and object occurs rather late in the grand scheme of things. And Winnicott is very clear that, until such a developmental stage has been attained, there is no such capacity.

Winnicott, therefore, suggests that the recognition of separateness between self and object must precede internalization; Kohut, on the other hand, suggests that internalization is an important part of the process by which the separateness between self and object becomes established.

Given these two rather different models, how do we conceptualize the relationship between the capacity to internalize and the recognition of separateness between self and object? I would like to propose a way to integrate the two theories. Kohut says that the selfobject is experienced as a part of the self; more accurately, perhaps, the selfobject that gratifies is experienced as a part of the self. As long as the object is experienced as an extension of the self, there is nothing that needs to be mastered and no impetus for internalization.

It is only when the selfobject frustrates that it is experienced (at least momentarily) as separate from the self. In fact, the experience of disappointment in the selfobject is an important part of what establishes the object as outside one's sphere of influence, as separate from the self. Then, once the object is experienced as external to the self, it can be internalized—in order to preserve it.

As the functions performed by the selfobject are internalized, the self no longer needs the object to function as a selfobject and can more easily accept the fact of the object's separateness.

And so frustration is a reminder of the separateness between self and object; it provides the impetus for internalizations that then make possible acceptance of the actual separateness between self and object.

WHAT IS A DISRUPTED POSITIVE TRANSFERENCE?

The therapist, then, does the best he can to understand the patient's need for narcissistic gratification and to resonate empathically with such need. And when he senses that the patient must have actual gratification, the therapist does the best he can to comply with the patient's need for direct gratification.

But inevitably the therapist does fail the patient. The self-cohesiveness of the patient and the stability of the selfobject transference will be momentarily disrupted, temporarily threatened.

The therapist's failure is experienced as a narcissistic injury, and the patient's reaction is one of outrage, devastation, and a regressive retreat.

WHAT IS NARCISSISTIC RAGE?

The narcissistic patient experiences rage whenever he feels that his will has been thwarted; and, in the aftermath of a narcissistic injury, the patient insists that he get recompense, insists that it be made up to him somehow. He has an abiding conviction that he is entitled to compensation in the here and now for damage sustained early on.

When the selfobject therapist commits an empathic failure, the patient is upset with the selfobject for having failed to perform its assigned function and for having demonstrated its fallibility, the fact of its limitations. The patient alternates between enraged protests at his own imperfection and angry reproaches against the therapist for having permitted the insult.

Narcissistic rage is a so-called breakdown, or disintegration, product of selfobject failure. There is an important difference between narcissistic rage and anger/aggression. Whereas anger and aggression are the reactions of a healthy self to frustration, rage is the reaction of a damaged self.

Healthy anger is directed not against objects (experienced as separate from the self) but against selfobjects (experienced as necessary to complete the self). Aggression in the healthy self, then, is mobilized in response to frustration and its purpose is to remove whatever barriers may be interfering with the gratification of a particular need or the pursuit of a particular goal. Howard and Margaret Baker (1987) have suggested that "we may get angry at a recalcitrant nail that will not go into a wall when we try to hang a picture. However, when the nail finally yields and the picture is hung, the anger subsides" (p. 6).

On the other hand, if the nail provokes a narcissistic injury and makes us feel defective or flawed, we may become enraged and attempt to retaliate against the nail, by slamming it into the wall. Even then, the rage may persist. Narcissistic rage seeks revenge; it pushes us to get even, often without caring about the resultant damage (done either to the self or to the object).

HOW DOES THE THERAPIST LOCATE THE OFFENDING FAILURE?

When the therapist, despite his best efforts, inadvertently fails the patient, an empathic rupture occurs and we speak of the positive transference as having been disrupted.

In the aftermath of the therapist's failure of the patient, the therapist directs his efforts toward identifying the offending failure. The work involves a focus not upon the legitimacy of the patient's upset but rather upon an understanding of the precipitating event that led to the patient's withdrawal. It is not the regressive position itself but the need for the retreat that should be the focus of the therapist's attention.

A correct identification by the therapist of the exact nature of the offending failure, no matter how minor, will be necessary if the failure is to afford the opportunity for internalization and structural growth.

To pinpoint the offending failure, the therapist may ask, "How have I let you down?" or " How have I failed you?" The emphasis is not on the patient's pathology. The question is not "How do you feel that I have disappointed you?" but rather "How have I disappointed you?" The reality is that the therapist, by being less than perfect, has indeed disappointed the patient. Given that the patient had imagined that he had finally found the good (perfect) parent he had never had, of course he is now devastated and outraged by the therapist's demonstration of his fallibility.

WHAT IS REQUIRED OF THE THERAPIST?

If the therapist has his own unresolved narcissistic issues and has not yet transformed his need to be perfectly empathic into a capacity to tolerate being imperfectly empathic (that is, sometimes unempathic), then each time he fails the patient, he will be unable to tolerate the patient's disenchantment with him. And if the therapist has secretly shared the patient's fantasy that he, the therapist, can and should be the perfect parent who will be able to make up the difference to the patient, then the therapist will find intolerable the patient's devastation, outrage, and accusations of betrayal.

In other words, the therapist must be able to tolerate his own lack of perfection; if the therapist cannot accept his own imperfection, then he cannot possibly expect the patient to come to terms with imperfection — whether in his contemporary objects, the transference object, the infantile object, or the patient himself.

How many therapists, in response to a patient's enraged protest that the therapist has been unempathic or that the therapist simply does not understand, have the capacity to feel good about themselves even as they are admitting that perhaps, in this particular instance, they were unempathic or didn't understand?

In demonstrating his fallibility, the therapist really has let the patient down; and he needs to be able to hear the patient out, without suffering too severe a blow to his own self-esteem. The patient is not distorting; the patient, in discovering the therapist's limitations, is accurately perceiving him as imperfect.

Together, patient and therapist confront the reality of how limited the therapist really is — and grieve it. Would that the therapist could always be empathic and attuned, compassionate and concerned. Would that the therapist were never demanding or impatient, critical or insistent. Would that the therapist could simply make the patient better by giving him now what he never had in a consistent, reliable way early on. Would that the therapist could heal the patient's wounds by way of the therapist's understanding and love. Patient and therapist must both come to terms with the sad reality of the therapist's limitations.

IS MISPERCEPTION INVOLVED IN THE PATIENT'S UPSET WITH THE THERAPIST?

When the patient experiences the therapist as having failed him, the patient is, then, accurately perceiving the therapist as imperfect, limited, fallible. The patient's disenchantment arises in the context of his realistic perception of the therapist as less perfect, more flawed, than he had originally envisioned. He had needed the therapist to be perfect; as part of the work he must do to master the thwarting of his desire, he must confront the reality of his disillusionment—and grieve it.

But the situation will be complicated if, in the aftermath of the therapist's empathic failure of him, the patient's pathogenic introjects (internal records of the parental badness) are activated and projected onto the therapist. Now a situation in which the therapist was being accurately perceived as less good than the patient had wanted him to be becomes transformed into a situation in which the therapist is being inaccurately perceived as bad. In other words, the disrupted positive transference (involving realistic perception of the therapist as disappointing) will be eclipsed by the concurrent presence of a negative transference (involving misperception—distorted perception—of the therapist as traumatically disappointing).

When both disrupted positive transference and negative transference exist simultaneously, an empathic failure that might otherwise have been experienced as a nontraumatic frustration becomes a traumatic frustration—that is, a traumatic recapitulation of the early-on traumatic failure situation. The negative transference must be worked through before the patient can grieve the loss of his illusions about the therapist as the perfect parent he never had.

In summary, whereas negative transference involves inaccurate perception (distortion) and positive transference involves inaccurate perception (illusion), disrupted positive transference (uncomplicated by the concurrence of negative transference) involves accurate perception, realistic perception of the therapist as less perfect than the patient had imagined him to be.

IS NOT THE POSITIVE TRANSFERENCE A SITUATION OF SEDUCTION AND BETRAYAL?

In a way, sleight of hand is involved. On the one hand, we encourage the patient with impaired capacity and structural deficit to deliver his infantile needs into the transference; we imply that it will be safe for him to have such expectations in relation to us. We do not interpret his need to have us be perfect. We allow it to be, implying that we are comfortable with being experienced that way and potentially capable of gratifying his need for perfection. In essence, we seduce him into having all sorts of magical expectations about us.

On the other hand, once the patient has finally developed a full-blown narcissistic transference, he finds that we periodically disappoint him, that we are not perfect, and that we cannot always deliver what he had thought we could. In other words, we betray him; and we do it repeatedly.

How can this be right? Is it fair to offer the promise of something and then fail to deliver? It is perhaps the ultimate seduction and betrayal, to imply that we will be able to gratify the patient's infantile expectations and then to disappoint him over and over again, when it turns out that we really are so very imperfect.

By way of an answer, I would like to propose the following: When the child's developmental needs are repeatedly and traumatically frustrated, he eventually represses them, so that he will not have to be in the position of having his heart broken again and again. As long as his needs are buried, we have no access to them, because the system is a closed one. Only with the therapeutic remobilization of his thwarted needs and their delivery into the transference can we convert a system that had once been closed into an open system to which we now have access.

Yes, as the therapist of someone who needs us to be perfect, we will be in the position of disappointing the patient over and over again, because we are not perfect. That perception is realistic, not unrealistic.

But if each such disappointment is the occasion for grieving the therapist's nontraumatic failures and the parent's traumatic failures, then we will be helping the patient come to terms with reality — the reality of the therapist's nontoxic failures and the parent's toxic failures of the patient.

Heartache and disappointment recapitulated in the transference will afford the patient an opportunity for the reworking of heartache and disappointment experienced at the hands of the parent. It will enable the patient to reexperience the original devastation, to put it into words and into perspective, to learn to bear it, and eventually to move on.

As we know, part of mastering the pain of the disillusionment are the defensive and adaptive internalizations that occur during that grieving process. Transmuting internalization and accretion of internal psychic structure result from the experience of having had and then lost.

Unless the patient has had the opportunity to have illusions about the therapist, to lose them, and to work those losses through, there is no such opportunity for structural growth, no such opportunity for the adding of new good. And the patient with impaired capacity and structural deficit will be destined always to be yearning for something he can never have, destined forever to be feeling empty, impoverished, and alone, destined always to be in pursuit of what he cannot have.

So there is, admittedly, an initial seduction and then repeated betrayals, but it is the recovery from such betrayals that constitutes the working-through process and is the means by which the patient is enabled to do some belated grieving and structure building. As he develops capacity, he lets go of his illusions, illusions he has clung to in order not to have to feel his pain.

HOW IS THE DISILLUSIONMENT STATEMENT USEFUL?

The working-through process is a process of gradual disillusionment; as such, it is a prolonged grieving process. The disillusionment statement can be used to help the patient access his grief about the therapist's nontoxic failure of him and, before that, his parent's toxic failure of him.

In the first part of the disillusionment statement, the therapist highlights the patient's illusions about the therapist's perfection. In the second part, the therapist empathically resonates with the patient's experience of disillusionment, disappointment at the discovery of the therapist's imperfection.

Disillusionment statements facilitate the working through of disrupted positive transferences; they facilitate the grieving the patient must do to let go of his illusions.

Examples of disillusionment statements:

> "You had thought that I would be able to help you recover some memories of the early abuse, but I haven't been able to do that and you find yourself feeling hurt and disappointed."

> "You had thought that it was not unreasonable to be expecting that you would be feeling much better by now, and it upsets you

THE POSITIVE TRANSFERENCE AND ITS DISRUPTIONS

to be realizing that, even after some years, you still feel depressed much of the time."

"You were so hoping that I would give you a hug, and it angers you that I won't."

"You were so hoping that I would be able to help you find a boyfriend, and it upsets that I have not been able to do that."

"All you were wanting was a little advice, and it's frustrating for you that I haven't offered you that."

HOW IS THE INTEGRATION STATEMENT USEFUL?

In the aftermath of the therapist's disillusionment of the patient, when the patient is feeling so devastated by the therapist's failure of him that he cannot remember ever having felt good about the therapist, integration statements may be useful.

Examples of integration statements:

"When you are feeling this upset, it is hard to remember that you ever had faith in me."

"When you are feeling this angry, it is difficult to keep in mind that you ever cared about me."

"When you are feeling this angry, it is difficult to remember that I care about you."

"When you are feeling this disappointed, you have trouble remembering that you used to look forward to coming because it felt so good to be here."

"When you are hurting as you are now, it is a struggle to remember why you would want to keep living."

Integration statements facilitate the patient's working through of his bad feelings about someone he had once experienced as good.

WHAT MUST THE PATIENT GRIEVE?

The therapist's present failure recreates for the patient the parent's early-on failure of him as a child. Although the parent's failures were toxic and intolerably horrid and the therapist's failures are nontoxic and not so horrid, being failed by someone who has come to mean the world to him (as once his parent did and now his therapist does) revives for the patient all the old hurt, the old pain, the old outrage.

In the associative material, the patient may recover significant childhood memories and genetic reconstructions may be possible.

The patient rants, raves, sobs, wails, weeps, screams out his anguish and his pain and his outrage. Interestingly, it is in the context of being held by the therapist that the patient can now let himself feel, in the present, in the context of his current disillusionment, his grief—grief that belongs more to the parent who traumatically failed the child than to the therapist who is now nontraumatically failing the patient.

In other words, devastation reexperienced in the relationship with the therapist offers the patient an opportunity to rework the original devastation. Belatedly, he grieves the early-on privations, deprivations, and insults.

On behalf of the child he once was, the patient grieves the reality of just how unspeakably horrid the parent was; on his own behalf now, the patient grieves the reality of the therapist's very real limitations and inadequacies. The patient gets it, deep within him, that he is ultimately powerless to do anything to make those realities any different, much as he might have wished to be able to do so. Genuine grieving, as we know, involves confronting the reality of just how bad it really was and is; and it means coming to terms with that, knowing there is nothing now that can be done to change it.

The patient begins to get it that his objects may not always be exactly as he would have wanted them to be; he grieves the lack of perfection within the therapist, within his parents, within his significant other, within his children, within the world, and within himself. He would have wanted things to be otherwise, and it pains him terribly that they are as they are. But he begins to make his peace with this. As Kopp (1969) writes, "Genuine grief is the sobbing and wailing which express the acceptance of our helplessness to do anything about losses" (p. 30).

HOW IS PARADOX INVOLVED?

Paradoxically, as the patient confronts the reality that he will not be able to be made better simply by way of the therapist's provision of perfect parenting, he internalizes the good parenting that the therapist really has been able to offer and, in the process, develops the capacity to provide for himself that good parenting. As he masters his disappointment with the limitations in the therapist's parenting of him, he internalizes what good there has been in that relationship and becomes, for himself, a good parent. In grieving the good that wasn't (and the bad that was), the patient is able to develop internal resources and capacity. As Kopp (1969) writes, "By no longer refusing to mourn the loss of the parents whom he wished for but never had, he can get to keep whatever was really there for him" (p. 33).

The patient gradually replaces his illusion that the therapist will be for him the good parent he never had with a reality—namely, that he will have to become for himself the good parent he never had. His need for illusion gets replaced by a capacity to tolerate reality.

WHAT IS INVOLVED IN GRIEVING HIS DISENCHANTMENT?

It is the work of grieving, the constant, repetitive raging, screaming, sobbing, and wailing, that is the process whereby the patient gradually lets go of his illusions.

Grieving is the way in which structural growth occurs. It involves working through disruptions of the positive transference, working through disillusionment.

In other words, nontraumatic frustration, or optimal disillusionment, provides the impetus for internalizing a good object, more specifically, provides the impetus for internalizing the regulatory functions that the selfobject had been performing prior to its failure of the patient. Such internalizations are part of the grieving process and are the way the patient masters his experience of being failed.

In essence, when the object (be it the selfobject parent or the selfobject therapist) has been good and is then bad, the child/patient deals with his disappointment in the frustrating object by taking in the good that had been there prior to the introduction of the bad—so that he can preserve internally a piece of the original experience of external goodness.

Transmuting internalization and accretion of internal structure result from the experience of having had and then lost. Transmuting internalization enables the patient to make internal what had once been external, enables the patient, ultimately, to do for himself what he had once needed from his objects.

And so it is that the patient is gradually able to give up the illusions he has clung to in order not to have to feel his pain. As the illusions are relinquished, the resistance is overcome. The patient's need to experience his objects as the good/perfect parent he never had becomes transformed into a capacity to provide for himself such parenting and, therefore, to tolerate the reality that his objects will not always be as good/perfect as he would have wanted them to be. As the patient becomes for himself the good parent he never had, his need to have his objects be perfect becomes transformed into a capacity to accept them as they are—imperfect, to be sure, but nonetheless plenty good enough.

More generally, the need to experience reality as other (better) than it is becomes transformed into a capacity to experience it as it really is, uncontaminated by the past. Such a process of transformation is accompanied by the taming of need, the internalization of function, the accretion of structure, and the development of capacity. Where once there was need, now there is capacity. Self psychology helps us to understand this developmental process by which infantile need is transformed into mature capacity.

HOW DO SELF PSYCHOLOGISTS CONCEIVE OF MENTAL HEALTH?

For the self psychologists, then, growing up (the task of the child) and getting better (the task of the patient) have to do with learning to master the disenchantment that comes with the recognition of just how imperfect the world is. Moving from infantile need to mature capacity has to do with mastering the loss of illusions about the perfection or the perfectability of the world. It has to do with transforming the need for one's objects to be other than, better than, who they are into the capacity to accept them as they are.

ELEVEN

The Negative Transference

WHY DO WE TURN FROM SELF PSYCHOLOGY TO OBJECT RELATIONS THEORY IN ORDER TO UNDERSTAND THE NEGATIVE TRANSFERENCE AND ITS RESOLUTION?

In the previous chapter, we explored the contributions of self psychology to our understanding of how psychic structure gets laid down or mapped out. I suggest that self psychology provides a more comprehensive model for understanding structural growth than does either classical psychoanalysis or object relations theory.

But although self psychology offers an excellent model for the addition of new good structure, it does little to improve our understanding of how old bad structure is modified. Self psychology is, after all, a theory about structural deficit, not relational conflict; absence of good, not presence of bad; the filling in of deficit, not the resolution of conflict. There are no internal bad objects or pathogenic introjects in self theory—only impaired or absent capacity.

To repeat, self psychology is a theory about the internal absence of good; it is not a theory about the internal presence of bad. Its interest is in the internal recording and structuralizing of good experiences, not the internal recording and structuralizing of bad experiences; it offers us, therefore, a theory about structural growth, not structural change.

It is to object relations theory, whose building blocks are internal bad objects, that we must look in order to understand both how pathogenic structures get there to begin with and how such structures, once there, can be modified—a process of structural change that involves working through the negative transference.

WHY IS THE DISTINCTION BETWEEN THE ABSENCE OF GOOD AND THE PRESENCE OF BAD SO IMPORTANT?

It is important to remember that, when we are talking about the internal absence of good (in the sense of missing structure and impaired capacity), the patient must be given the opportunity to deliver his need for external good into the transference. Gradual internalization of the good encountered there is the process by which the internal absence of good is corrected for.

The deficiency-compensation model of therapeutic action conceives of the therapeutic relationship as offering the patient a chance to start over, an opportunity to begin anew.

But when we are talking about the internal presence of bad (in the form of internal bad objects or pathogenic introjects that are the internal records of the early-on traumas), it is not enough that the patient have the experience of external good and an opportunity to internalize it—because the internal toxicity will still be there.

Rather, the patient must be given the opportunity to modify the bad that already exists. In other words, when the patient's traumatic history has been permanently recorded in the form of toxic internal structures, the patient must have the chance to modify the bad that is already inside (by detoxifying those pathogenic structures). The patient is able to rework the internalized badness by experiencing first "old bad" in the relationship with the therapist and then "bad made good." This is the process by which the internal presence of bad is corrected for.

The relational-conflict model of therapeutic action conceives of the therapeutic relationship as offering the patient this chance for belated mastery, this opportunity to rework the original traumas.

WHAT IS THE RELATIONSHIP BETWEEN STRUCTURAL GROWTH AND STRUCTURAL CHANGE?

Whereas structural growth involves structural deficit, structural change involves relational conflict.

Whereas structural growth involves the addition of new good, structural change involves the modification of old bad.

Whereas structural growth is effected by way of working through disruptions of the positive transference, structural change is effected by way of working through the negative transference.

Whereas the patient's need for the good parent he never had makes structural growth possible, the patient's need for the bad parent he did have makes structural change possible.

Whereas structural growth involves transformation of the infantile need for illusion into the capacity to experience reality as it is, structural change involves transformation of the infantile need for distortion into the capacity to experience reality as it is.

Whereas we turn to self psychology to help us conceptualize the process of structural growth (be it with respect to the drive structures of classical psychoanalysis or the self structures of self psychology), we turn to object relations theory to help us conceptualize the process of structural change.

WHAT ARE CLINICAL EXAMPLES OF STRUCTURAL GROWTH?

Let us think about different situations (of positive transference) that involve the patient's relentless pursuit of infantile gratification in the treatment situation. Into what capacity is the infantile need for a good parent transformed by way of working through disruptions of the positive transference?

1. With respect to the patient's neurotic (oral) need to consume: transformation of rapacious hunger into a more modulated appetite.
2. With respect to the patient's neurotic (anal) need to oppose: transformation of stubborn oppositionalism into a more tempered assertiveness.
3. With respect to the patient's narcissistic need for validation: transformation of the need for external reinforcement into a capacity to provide such reinforcement internally.
4. With respect to the patient's narcissistic need for perfection: transformation of the relentless pursuit of perfection into a capacity to tolerate imperfection.

WHAT ARE CLINICAL EXAMPLES OF STRUCTURAL CHANGE?

Let us think about different situations (of negative transference) that involve the patient's compulsive need to re-create the early-on traumatic failure situation in the relationship with the therapist. Into what capacity is the infantile need for a bad object transformed by way of working through the negative transference?

1. With respect to the patient's compulsive need to re-create in the transference the dynamic of victimization: transformation of both his need to experience the therapist as abusive and his need to be abusive (to the therapist and to himself) into a capacity to assert himself.
2. With respect to the patient's compulsive need to re-create in the transference the dynamic of criticism: transformation of both his need to experience the therapist as critical and his need to be critical (of the therapist and of himself) into a capacity to be more realistic in his appraisals.
3. With respect to the patient's compulsive need to re-create in the transference the dynamic of unrealistic expectations:

transformation of both his need to experience the therapist as relentlessly demanding and his need to be relentlessly demanding (of the therapist and of himself) into a capacity to be more accepting.

WHAT ACCOMPANIES THESE TRANSFORMATIONS?

As the patient's transferential need for the good parent is transformed into healthy capacity by way of structural growth and his transferential need for the bad parent is transformed into healthy capacity by way of structural change, the patient develops an ability to harness his energy so that it empowers him, enabling him to provide for himself where once he needed the object to provide for him and enabling him to move forward in his life toward the realization of his potential and his dreams, both personal and professional.

WHAT ARE THE THERAPEUTIC AGENTS OF CHANGE?

In the literature, numerous papers have been written about the so-called therapeutic action of psychodynamic psychotherapy, in other words, what is it about the therapeutic process that is healing?

Those who espouse a one-person theory of therapeutic action believe that insight by way of interpretation (particularly the transference interpretation) is the primary therapeutic agent. Classical psychoanalysis is, of course, a prime example of such a perspective.

The therapeutic aim is thought to be a strengthening of the ego, an extending of its province such that it can deal more effectively with id pressure from below and superego pressure from above. As the ego becomes stronger by way of the insight it acquires, its defenses become less necessary. As the defenses are gradually relinquished, the patient becomes less conflicted (less neurotic) and we speak of the patient's conflict as having been resolved. Achievement of insight makes possible the resolution of conflict. This is described in the classical literature as a conflict-resolution model.

Those who espouse a two-person theory of therapeutic action believe that it is the relationship itself between patient and therapist that ultimately heals the patient — a corrective experience provided by way of the real relationship that ultimately effects the cure.

As we discussed in a previous chapter, two-person theories of therapeutic action conceive of the therapeutic setting in two different ways. Those who believe in a deficiency-compensation model (as do most self psychologists) emphasize the role of the therapist as offering the patient an opportunity to experience something new and good; those who believe in a relational-conflict model (as do many object relations theorists) emphasize the role of the therapist as offering the patient an opportunity to experience something old and bad. Although this latter model involves an initial reexperiencing of the therapist as the old bad object, in the final analysis it is the fact that the therapist is a new good object that the damage the patient sustained early on is ultimately corrected for.

In both two-person models, therefore, it is in the context of the new relationship between patient and therapist that there is the opportunity for correction of the original environmental failure situation, the new relationship a corrective for the old one.

In summary, with respect to the curative agent, a one-person theory focuses upon insight and a two-person theory focuses upon the real relationship. By the same token, a one-person theory emphasizes the gaining of knowledge and a two-person theory emphasizes the provision of experience.

HOW DOES THE THERAPIST INTERVENE WHEN INSIGHT IS THE GOAL? HOW DOES HE INTERVENE WHEN A CORRECTIVE EXPERIENCE IS THE GOAL?

If the provision of insight is the goal, then the therapist's interventions should direct the patient's attention inward and backward (to the past) so that he will be able to observe his internal process and the fact of his unconscious repetitions, his tendency to experience new objects as old ones. The net result, as we discussed earlier, is a strengthening of the ego and increased self-awareness.

If the provision of a corrective experience is the goal, then the therapist's interventions should direct the patient's attention outward so that he will be able to observe and experience the reality of who the therapist is in the here and now. The therapist is a new good object, not the old bad one, and the therapist wants the patient ultimately to feel that and to profit from it. The net result, as we discussed earlier, is compensation for the early-on environmental failures.

I believe that an integrative approach to the patient that combines both a one-person perspective (with its emphasis on insight) and a two-person perspective (with its emphasis on the relationship itself) will be maximally effective. More specifically, combining both perspectives works particularly well when a patient is in the throes of a negative transference.

Therefore, to facilitate resolution of a negative transference, the therapist must strive both to enhance the patient's knowledge of himself and to provide a corrective experience.

HOW IS INSIGHT A CORRECTIVE FOR TRANSFERENCE DISTORTION?

Negative transference is a case of mistaken identity; the patient mistakenly perceives the therapist as the old bad object. (Again, as noted in an earlier chapter, our focus here will be upon those situations that involve unrealistic perceptions of, or inappropriate reactions to, the therapist. In what follows, we will be less concerned with those situations in which the therapist unwittingly participates with the patient in his dramatic reenactments — unless the discussion is about a situation of projective identification.)

When insight is thought to be the corrective, the therapist, in order to correct the patient's distortion, offers interpretations that direct the patient's attention inward and backward, encouraging him to observe his internal process and his tendency to make (negative) assumptions about the present based on the past, in other words, his tendency to have (negative) expectations about new good objects, including the therapist, based on bad experiences with old ones.

The therapist does not specifically address the reality of the current situation, does not specifically suggest that the patient's perceptions of him are wrong. The therapist simply calls the patient's attention to the fact that the patient does seem to expect, unconsciously, that his current objects will fail him in the very same ways that the infantile object had failed him.

The message to the patient, whether explicit or implicit, is: "You tend always to make the assumption that your objects, including me, will be just the way your (bad) parent was. Interesting, yes?" The patient is being encouraged to observe his internal process and to become aware of the recurrence of certain themes in his interactions with others. He is gaining an appreciation of the extent to which his perceptions of reality are contaminated by his compulsive need to experience the present in ways determined by his unresolved past.

The result is the rendering conscious of what had been unconscious, increased self-awareness, and a strengthening of the ego. In other words, the patient gains a better understanding of all the ways in which he organizes his experience of himself and his world around the toxic interactions he had early on.

The acquisition of such insight will, therefore, be part of what motivates the patient ultimately to relinquish the transference distortion.

HOW IS THE RELATIONSHIP ITSELF A CORRECTIVE FOR TRANSFERENCE DISTORTION?

When the real relationship is thought to be the corrective, the therapist, in order to correct the patient's distortion, offers interpretations that direct the patient's attention outward, encourage him to experience the reality of who the therapist actually is in the here and now — namely, that he is a new good object, not the old bad one.

Now the therapist does address the reality of the current situation. The therapist challenges the patient's distortion (challenges the patient's unconscious projection) by confronting the patient with the reality of who he, the therapist, actually is.

The message to the patient, whether explicit or implicit, is "I want you to see that I am not the bad person your parent was (and that you were therefore expecting me to be)." The patient is being encouraged to recognize that there is a discrepancy between what he had imagined was real and what is in fact real, a discrepancy between distortion on the one hand and reality on the other. A wedge is being created between the patient's subjective experience of the therapist as the old bad object and the objective reality of the therapist as a new good object.

The result is the creation of tension within the patient between what he is coming to know (informed by positive experience with the therapist in the present) and what he had been assuming (informed by negative experience with the parent in the past).

Ultimately, the patient must let go of the transference distortion because of his need to reconcile what he comes to experience as real with what he had feared was real; in other words, he relinquishes the distortion because of his need to integrate his new (reality-based) experience of the therapist as a good object with his old (distortion-based) experience of the therapist as a bad object.

The relationship itself between patient and therapist will, therefore, be part of what motivates the patient ultimately to relinquish the transference distortion.

HOW IS PARADOX INVOLVED?

The transference distortion is relinquished, then, when the patient can recognize the split between his experience of the therapist as an old bad object (which is informed by his past) and his knowledge of the therapist as a new good object (which is informed by the present).

There is, however, a paradox involved here: It is only as the patient becomes able to experience the therapist as he really is that the therapist can truly become available as a new object. On the other hand, it is because the therapist is a new object that the patient gradually becomes able to experience the therapist as he really is.

Just as a sculptor chips away at a block of granite, exposing underneath the true form of his sculpture, so too patient and therapist work together to chip away at the patient's misperceptions of the therapist to expose the underlying form of the therapist. It is then that the therapist truly becomes available to the patient as a new object, as someone who can offer the patient an actual experience in the here and now that will be a corrective. And it is then that we can speak of the real relationship as having the potential to correct for the transference distortions; as the distortions are gradually chipped away, the therapist becomes available as a new good object.

HOW DOES OBJECT RELATIONS THEORY INFORM OUR UNDERSTANDING OF HOW THE NEGATIVE TRANSFERENCE IS RESOLVED?

To this point, we have been looking at how the patient lets go of distorted perceptions of the therapist because of both the insight he acquires about his tendency to repeat the old in the new and the actual experience he has of being in relationship with the therapist. The emphasis has been upon how insight and experience can, at any particular point in time, challenge the patient's distorted experience of the therapist.

Let us look now at what happens over time, at how actual structural change is effected in the underlying pathogenic structures that fuel the patient's distortions and the negative transference. We will look to object relations theory, particularly the contributions of Klein (1964, 1975), to inform our understanding of how modifications of the structural configuration of the patient's internal world are actually accomplished.

Object relations theory conceives of the (negative) transference in a dynamic sense as involving a series of cycles of projection and introjection. From this perspective, one can envision a working-through process that requires a number of steps and a series of interactions (between patient and therapist) through which a pathogenic introject must pass before it is gradually detoxified and assimilated as healthy capacity.

The working-through process goes as follows. The patient, under the sway of the repetition compulsion, projects a pathogenic introject onto the therapist, who is then experienced as the old bad parent (projection) or actually made to become the old bad parent (projective identification). In other words, the patient may either experience the therapist, in a distorted fashion, as the old bad parent or, by way of exerting interpersonal pressure on the therapist to accept his projection, actually make the therapist (at least momentarily) into the old bad object; in this latter instance, we speak of the therapist as initially and unwittingly accepting the patient's projection.

But the therapist is not, in point of fact, the old bad object at all—but a new good one. Ultimately, the therapist challenges the patient's projection by lending aspects of his otherness (or, as Winnicott [1965] would say, his "externality") to the interaction—so that the patient will be able to have the experience of something that is "other-than-me" and can then take that in.

The patient must both understand and experience the difference between what he had expected (fueled by negative past experience) and what actually happens. The patient must both recognize with his head and experience with his heart the fact that the therapist is a new good object.

What is then internalized is an amalgam, part contributed by the therapist and part contributed by the patient (the original projection); in other words, part is new and good, part is old and bad.

By the same token, what gets projected the next time around is a little less toxic, a little more reality-based. And what gets introjected on each successive round is ever less distorted. By way of a series of such microinternalizations, the patient's pathogenic introjects are gradually reworked, rendered less toxic.

In essence, it is by way of ongoing and repetitive serial dilutions that the patient's underlying pathogenic introjects are gradually modified in the direction of reality. With each successive cycle of projection (by the patient of the pathogenic introject onto the therapist), challenge (by the therapist of the pathogenic introject), and reintrojection (by the patient of the now-slightly-modified-in-the-direction-of-reality introject), the pathogenic introject is gradually detoxified.

The cycle is repeated again and again, each time the pathogenic structure becoming a little less toxic.

As the underlying introjects become more reality-based, the patient's perceptions become more accurate, and we speak eventually of the negative transference as having been resolved. Whereas once the patient had needed to experience the therapist as the bad parent he had, now the patient develops the capacity to experience the therapist more realistically, as he actually is.

It is this working-through process that enables the patient to master the original trauma and to transform the internalized badness into healthy structure and capacity.

I am suggesting, therefore, that the process of effecting deep change involves ongoing interactive cycles between patient and therapist — and object relations theory informs our understanding of this dynamic.

HOW DO WE RECOGNIZE THE EXISTENCE OF A NEGATIVE TRANSFERENCE?

A negative transference unfolds when the patient delivers, by way of projection, his internal bad objects (or pathogenic introjects) into the treatment situation and the interactional dynamic that had existed between the patient and his parent is recreated in the transference between the patient and the therapist. The patient now experiences the therapist, in a distorted fashion, as the bad parent he had or may fear that, at some point in the future, the therapist will turn out to be the bad parent he had. Both situations speak to negative transference, whether the badness is experienced in the present or expected in the future.

WHAT IS THE RELATIONSHIP BETWEEN PROJECTION AND TRANSFERENCE ON THE ONE HAND AND PROJECTIVE IDENTIFICATION AND COUNTERTRANSFERENCE ON THE OTHER?

Whereas projection relates to the transference, projective identification relates to the countertransference as well. In other words, when projection is involved and the patient is simply imagining that the therapist is the bad object, then the therapist can intervene in ways that highlight the conflict within the patient between his knowledge of reality (informed by the present) and his experience of reality (informed by the past). But when projective identification is involved

THE NEGATIVE TRANSFERENCE

and the therapist is participating (countertransferentially) with the patient in the latter's dramatic reenactments, then the situation is much more complicated.

Let us now consider both direct transference (which involves usually projection and much less often projective identification) and inverted transference (which involves usually projective identification and much less often simply projection).

HOW DO DIRECT TRANSFERENCE, PROJECTION, AND PROJECTIVE IDENTIFICATION RELATE TO ONE ANOTHER?

Let us consider a situation of direct transference involving projection. When the patient projects the bad parent introject onto the therapist (and the therapist refuses to accept it), we have a situation of direct transference. The patient experiences the therapist, in a distorted fashion, as the powerful, victimizing parent he once had and experiences himself, similarly in a distorted fashion, as the helpless, vulnerable child he once was. A direct transference recapitulates the early-on traumatic failure situation, with the therapist cast in the role of the victimizer and the patient assigned the role of the victim.

In such a situation, the therapist is not really a powerful victimizer and the patient is not really a powerless victim — although this is the patient's experience.

But let us think now about a situation of direct transference that involves not projection but projective identification.

When the patient projects the bad parent introject onto the therapist and exerts pressure on the therapist to become bad, we have a situation of projective identification — if the therapist accepts the projection. It happens less often that the patient is able to get the therapist to participate with him in his dramatic reenactment, but it certainly does happen.

The patient now experiences the therapist, in a realistic fashion, as the powerful, victimizing parent he once had and becomes himself the helpless, vulnerable child he once was. The early-on traumatic failure situation will have been replicated.

In such a situation of projective identification, the therapist becomes the powerful victimizer—the patient, his powerless victim.

IS PROJECTIVE IDENTIFICATION AN INSTANCE OF TRANSFERENCE?

We know that the transference involves a reexperiencing of the past in the present in a way that, as Greenson (1967) notes, "does not befit" (or "is inappropriate to") the present (p. 155). Transference always involves a misperceiving or a misinterpreting of the present in terms of the past.

So is projective identification an instance of transference? Well, yes and no. It is an instance of transference because it is created by way of the patient's inappropriate delivery of his infantile need to be failed into the treatment situation. But it is not an instance of transference because, once the therapist accepts the projection and participates with the patient in the latter's dramatic reenactment, the patient's perception of him as bad is no longer (transference) distortion but reality.

HOW DO INVERTED TRANSFERENCE, PROJECTION, AND PROJECTIVE IDENTIFICATION RELATE TO ONE ANOTHER?

When the patient (1) identifies with the powerful parent introject and (2) projects onto the therapist the powerless child introject, a scenario unfolds that is very different from the situation of a direct transference.

Let us imagine, for example, that the interactional dynamic between patient and therapist involves criticism—critical parent (with which the patient now identifies), criticized child (the position in which the patient places the therapist). Admittedly, it may be that the patient simply experiences himself as capable of being critical—but is not actually critical. Much more likely, however, is that the patient will feel critical of the therapist—and will actually be critical (expressing it more or less directly).

THE NEGATIVE TRANSFERENCE

Similarly, it is possible that the therapist will not experience himself as having been criticized. But it will be pretty hard to deny the reality that the patient is feeling/being critical of him. Much more likely, then, is that the therapist will feel criticized.

More generally, in a situation of inverted transference, usually both players participate in the dramatic reenactment and the situation is one that involves projective identification, with both patient and therapist actually assuming the roles assigned them. Inverted transference rarely involves, simply, projection.

In an inverted transference, then, the patient becomes in fact, and not just in fantasy, the actual bad parent and exerts pressure on the therapist to feel like the helpless, vulnerable child the patient once was. The patient, through his identification with the powerful, victimizing parent, relegates the therapist to a position of helplessness and vulnerability, the role the patient once had in relation to the parent. The therapist is thereby made to feel what it was really like for the child, growing up.

By way of inverted transference (and projective identification), the patient is able (usually unconsciously) to communicate to the therapist his internal experience of the toxic parent. The patient is able to get the therapist to understand, firsthand, just how awful it really was for him (the patient) as a child.

> **IN THIS CHAPTER ON NEGATIVE TRANSFERENCE, WHAT WILL OUR FOCUS BE?**

It is the situation of direct transference, wherein the patient experiences the therapist, in a distorted fashion, as like (or potentially like) the bad parent he actually had, that will be explored in this chapter. The situation that arises when the therapist is made into the bad (powerful) parent the patient once had and/or the bad (powerless) child the patient once was is beyond the scope of this primer. This situation involves projective identification (and/or inverted transference) and presents powerful opportunities for healing but requires use of the therapist's countertransferential reactions to inform the interventions he makes—which would take us well beyond our present focus on the transference and its resolution.

IN A NEGATIVE TRANSFERENCE, WHERE IS THE LOCUS OF CONTROL AND POWER?

In a situation of direct transference, the patient gives the therapist the control by projecting onto him the powerful parent introject. The therapist is able to be effective because, in a situation of direct transference, the patient vests the power in the therapist. Therefore, it should not be all that difficult for the therapist to facilitate resolution of the negative transference.

In a situation of inverted transference, however, the patient maintains the power, through his identification with the powerful parent and his assignment of powerlessness to the therapist (who will be hard-pressed not to accept such an assignment). In effect, the locus of control is invested in the patient, which robs the therapist of his therapeutic effectiveness and makes it much harder for the therapist to facilitate resolution of the negative transference. In other words, with a direct transference, the therapist retains his power. But with an inverted transference, the patient wrests the therapist's power from him and weakens him.

If the therapist, in such a situation, is to recover his therapeutic effectiveness and ability to provide, ultimately, a corrective influence, then he must find ways to intervene that will demonstrate his ability (1) to meet the patient's aggression, (2) to challenge the patient's provocativeness, and (3) to contain the patient's relentlessness—but, again, this takes us well beyond the scope of this primer.

WHAT ARE THE NEGATIVE FILTERS THROUGH WHICH THE PATIENT EXPERIENCES HIMSELF AND OTHERS?

The patient presents all kinds of unrealistically negative ideas about himself and his objects, deriving from early-on traumatic experiences internally recorded and structuralized as pathogenic structures. These introjects color and distort his perceptions of himself and, when projected, his perceptions of others. As a result, the patient has an abiding conviction that he is bad and/or his objects are bad.

To the extent that the patient continues to experience new good objects as old bad ones, to that extent will the patient be bound to his past, a slave to his unconscious repetitions, and blocked in his forward movement. To the extent that the patient continues to experience himself as defective, helpless, and incapable, to that extent will the patient be unable to take responsibility for his life and condemned instead to be forever perpetuating the status quo.

Our hope is that the patient, once he overcomes his resistance to engaging affectively with the therapist, will be able to deliver his internal toxicity into the treatment situation. Under the sway of the repetition compulsion, the patient will project onto the therapist the bad parent introject and a direct transference will unfold, in which the patient re-creates with the therapist the early-on traumatic failure situation and experiences the therapist as the bad parent he once had.

HOW IS THE DISTORTION STATEMENT USEFUL?

To facilitate resolution of the negative transference, the therapist offers interpretations that encourage the patient to observe the fact of his unconscious repetitions and to recognize that he tends to make assumptions about the present based on his unresolved past. By way of distortion statements that simply name, implying no judgment, the therapist strives to highlight the patient's unrealistically negative expectations about the therapist. The therapist wants to create a picture of the patient's (defensive) stance in relation to the therapist — and the world.

Examples of distortion statements:

"You are not sure that it is safe to talk about what most matters to you."

"You are concerned that I might use what you say against you."

"You are afraid that I will try to control you."

"Your fear is that I may be bored with you, not interested in what you have to say."

"You are afraid that I might laugh at you."

"You are afraid that I will misunderstand you as your mother did."

"You are reluctant to trust me for fear that I, like your father, will end up betraying you."

In a distortion statement, the therapist names the patient's fear, in an experience-near, nonjudgmental way, and/or attempts to highlight the connection between the patient's current fears and early-on negative experiences.

HOW IS THE LEGITIMIZATION STATEMENT USEFUL?

Earlier I suggested use of legitimization statements to contextualize both the longings that accompany a positive transference and the fears that accompany a negative transference. By way of a legitimization statement, the connection is specifically made between the past and the present; the negativity that the patient feels in relation to the therapist is framed as a legitimate response to early-on negative experience at the hands of the parent.

Examples of legitimization statements:

"Because your mother was relentlessly demanding, of course your fear is that I too will expect the impossible of you."

"Because your father was never satisfied with your performance, of course you find yourself feeling anxious that I too will be disappointed."

"Given that you never felt really safe as a child, of course you now find yourself feeling anxious, apprehensive, unsettled."

"Because you never felt understood as a child, of course your concern is that I too will be unable to appreciate who you really are."

"Because your mother would withdraw from you when she was angry, of course your fear is that I too will punish you by withholding my affection."

In each of these statements, the patient's current fear is understood against the backdrop of traumatic early-on experience. The patient's despair, anxiety, apprehensiveness, and distress are framed as understandable derivatives of childhood experiences never fully mastered and now delivered into the transference. The therapist is hoping that, by way of legitimization statements that both enhance the patient's knowledge of himself and validate his experience, the therapist will be able, in a gentle way, to deepen the patient's understanding of why he is as he is and what motivates him in his relationships.

HOW DOES THE THERAPIST DIRECT THE PATIENT'S ATTENTION INWARD AND BACKWARD?

The therapist uses distortion statements and legitimization statements to highlight, in a nonthreatening fashion, the presence of unrealistically negative misperceptions. The patient is not confronted with the reality of the situation; his distorted perceptions are not challenged. Rather, the therapist simply highlights the fact of the patient's unconscious repetitions. He does this by way of transference interpretations that direct the patient's attention inward and backward in order to observe his internal process and his tendency to experience new good objects as old bad ones.

HOW DOES THE ACHIEVEMENT OF INSIGHT FOSTER CHANGE?

The therapist wants the patient to recognize that he brings to his contemporary relationships ill-conceived ideas about himself and his objects that are not at all reality-based; they were internalized many, many years ago, are long since outdated, and are no longer functional at all.

The therapist hopes that the patient will come to understand not only the genetic origins of his distortions but also his investment in holding on to them, how having them serves him, and how much he pays for refusing to relinquish them.

As the patient becomes ever more aware of just how ill-founded his assumptions are, it will become increasingly difficult for him to maintain his attachment to the distortions that have for so long informed his experience of himself and his objects. In the face of increasingly clear evidence that what the patient had imagined to be real is at odds with what turns out to be real, it becomes harder and harder for the patient to remain attached to the past, denying the reality of the present situation.

HOW DOES THE THERAPIST DIRECT THE PATIENT'S ATTENTION OUTWARD?

In a one-person theory of therapeutic action, the patient is thought to relinquish his transference distortions as his ego gains more and more insight. But there is an equally powerful corrective provided by the relationship itself between patient and therapist—which two-person theories of therapeutic action inform us about. In other words, in addition to interventions (distortion and legitimization statements) that encourage the patient to look inward and backward in order to observe the fact of his unconscious repetitions, there are interventions (modification and inverted modification statements) that encourage the patient to look outward in order to experience the reality of who the therapist is.

With distortion and legitimization statements, the therapist names the patient's internal experience and carefully avoids addressing the external reality. Modification and inverted modification statements, however, focus more directly upon what is real in the patient's relationship with the therapist. By way of such statements, the therapist challenges the patient's unconscious projections by confronting the patient with the reality of who the therapist is. More accurately, by way of such statements, the therapist reminds the patient of what the patient really does know about the reality of who the therapist is (even if the patient chooses, sometimes, to forget).

Such interventions must be neither too threatening nor too anxiety-provoking or they will have defeated their purpose of opening the patient's eyes to the reality of who the therapist really is. The therapist must respect the patient's need to experience his new objects as old ones; the therapist must appreciate that the patient remains loyal to the infantile object and experiences any suggestion that things could now be (and therefore could once have been) different as a serious threat to his way of being in the world.

HOW CAN THE MODIFICATION STATEMENT BE USEFUL?

By way of a modification statement that places side by side the patient's knowledge of reality and his experience of it, the therapist strives to put a wedge between objective reality and the patient's subjective experience of it.

Like all conflict statements, the modification statement first names an anxiety-provoking reality that the patient, on some level, does know and then names the anxiety-assuaging defense (the distortion) to which the patient clings in order not to know. Like all conflict statements, the modification statement first directs the patient's attention to something that the patient would rather not be reminded of and then resonates with where the patient is.

Examples of modification statements:

1. "Even though you know that I take very seriously what you say, sometimes you find yourself holding back for fear that I might not appreciate just how important it really is to you."
2. "Although you know that I do not have expectations in here about what you should be doing, you find yourself feeling sometimes that I must be disappointed in you."
3. "Although you know that I am deeply committed to our work together, you find yourself worrying sometimes that maybe I am simply doing it for the money and don't really care."
4. "Even though you do know that I am very much with you, right now you find yourself feeling very alone and unsure of our connection—much as you must have felt in relation to your mother."
5. "Although you know that I do not judge you, you find yourself fearing that I, like your father, might."
6. "Even though you know that what you're doing feels right, there are times when you start to doubt yourself and your perceptions."
7. "Although you know that you do have some control over what happens to you, in the moment you are feeling particularly helpless and at a loss."

In the modification statements above, the therapist can emphasize different aspects of the tension within the patient between anxiety-provoking reality and anxiety-assuaging defense:

1. the therapist may simply highlight the internal tension within the patient between his knowledge of the therapist and his experience of him — which the first three interventions do;
2. the therapist may interpret more directly the patient's distorted experience of the therapist as a case of mistaken identity (the more appropriate culprit being the parent) — which the fourth and fifth interventions do; or
3. the therapist may emphasize not so much the patient's distorted perceptions of the therapist as powerfully victimizing but the patient's distorted perceptions of himself as helplessly inadequate and limited — which the sixth and seventh interventions do.

Whatever the focus, all modification statements remind the patient that the conflict is an internal one. Because the therapist wants to avoid struggling with the patient, he must not take it upon himself to be the voice of reality that challenges the patient's defensive need to feel what he feels and to do what he does.

In a modification statement, the therapist names a reality that challenges the patient's defense — but he names the reality as something that the patient knows, on some level, to be real. If the therapist uses his own voice to remind the patient of something that challenges the patient's perceptions, then the therapist will have made it more difficult for the patient to own what he knows to be real and to own that the conflict is an internal one. Furthermore, the therapist, by being himself the voice of reality, sets himself apart from the patient, who justifiably may then experience the therapist as having abandoned him at a time when he needed understanding.

HOW CAN THE INVERTED MODIFICATION STATEMENT BE USEFUL?

Whereas a modification statement speaks first to the force within the patient able to experience reality as it is and then to the force within

THE NEGATIVE TRANSFERENCE

the patient needing to deny that reality, an inverted modification statement speaks first to the patient's defense (which has now become the more anxiety-provoking side of his conflict) and then to the patient's capacity to know reality as it is (now the less anxiety-provoking side).

Inverted modification statements are addressed to a patient who is becoming more and more able to confront reality, uncontaminated by the need for it to be otherwise. Now it is more anxiety-provoking for the patient to be reminded of his fear (which ties him to the past) than it is for him to be reminded of reality (which is about the present).

Examples of inverted modification statements:

"Although sometimes you still feel overwhelmed and helpless, for the most part you are beginning to realize that how things turn out has to do with the choices you make."

"Although sometimes you get caught up in thinking that I (like your mother) don't appreciate just how hard it has been for you, you are starting to see that I do know how painful it has been and am very much with you in that."

"Even though you continue to feel, at times, that you have no control over what happens in here, it is much easier these days for you to remember that it is up to you to use your time in here in whatever ways you think will most benefit you."

"Although it makes you very anxious to admit it, you are beginning to think that you should try to remember whatever you can about your mother."

"Even though sometimes you get worried that I might be disappointed in you, for the most part you are able to remind yourself that I am not expecting you to perform for me in here. As you know, it was your father who had unrealistic expectations of you, not I."

Both modification and inverted modification statements are important tools for working through the negative transference. They challenge the patient's unconscious projections onto the therapist by juxtaposing what the patient really does know to be real, even if sometimes he chooses to forget, with what the patient fears is real.

WHAT HAPPENS AS THE PATIENT BEGINS TO EXPERIENCE THE THERAPIST AS A NEW GOOD OBJECT?

By way of a combination of insight and corrective experience, the patient is gradually enabled to feel, in the context of the real relationship with the therapist, that the therapist is a new good object and not the old bad one at all. As the patient comes to such a recognition, he is in a real bind. To remain attached to the infantile object is to deny the reality of the present situation, but to accept the reality of the present situation is to relinquish his ties to the past.

It becomes ever more difficult for the patient to maintain his attachment to his defenses (his distortions) in the face of increasingly clear evidence that what he had been assuming was real (based on negative experiences early on) is at odds with what he is coming to know as real (based on positive experiences in the here and now).

WHAT IS THE ROLE OF GRIEVING IN RESOLVING THE NEGATIVE TRANSFERENCE?

There comes a time, then, when the patient finally gets it that the therapist is truly different from the parent. That is, there comes a time when the patient can actually feel, in his relationship with the therapist, the difference between what's real and what's transferential.

In fact, the patient may never realize just how bad the parent really was until he has a new experience in the present that opens his eyes to just how bad it once was. As Clara Thompson (1950) has written, "In order to become conscious that something is wrong, one must have a new experience which makes one aware of new possibilities" (p. 105).

As the patient comes to understand what might have been, he begins to feel the horror of what was, and his heart breaks. He can no longer deny the reality of his heartache and his devastation. He grieves for the wounded child he once was and the damaged adult he then became. Belatedly he mourns, feeling, to the very depths of his soul, his anguish and his outrage about just how bad the parent really was, feeling now all the sorrow he could not possibly let himself experience as a child. Such is the work of grieving, such is the work of making one's peace with reality, and moving on.

As the patient grieves, the defenses become less and less necessary.

HOW DOES THE DEFENSE BECOME INCREASINGLY EGO-DYSTONIC?

Where once the defense, the pathology, was clung to in order to ease the anxiety the patient, as a child, would have felt had he let in the horrid reality of just how bad his parent really was, now the defense becomes itself a source of anxiety. Where once the defense served the patient by alleviating his anxiety, now the defense creates anxiety. Where once the defense was adaptive, now it is maladaptive; where once ego-syntonic, now ego-dystonic. As the patient gets more and more in touch with how maladaptive his defenses really are, the defenses not only serve him less and less well but also begin to create more and more anxiety. As the patient is more and more able to confront reality, the defenses becomes less and less necessary. By the same token, as the patient becomes less and less invested in his defenses, he becomes more and more able to confront reality.

WHAT IS THE ROLE OF THE SYNTHETIC FUNCTION OF THE EGO?

As the tension within the patient between his knowledge of reality and his experience of reality becomes ever greater, the synthetic function of the ego — whose goal is to promote integration — becomes ever more active in its efforts to reconcile the two elements in conflict, and the balance shifts in the direction of reality. Ultimately, the patient lets go of his distortions because of his need to integrate his knowledge of reality with his experience of it.

HOW DOES SEPARATION FROM THE INFANTILE OBJECT RELATE TO OVERCOMING THE RESISTANCE?

The patient's severing of his attachment to his distortions is accompanied by separation from the infantile object. As the patient gives up his investment in the infantile object, he lets go of his need for the transference object to be bad and relinquishes his need to be failed.

At this point, we speak of the negative transference as having been resolved and the resistance as having been overcome. The patient's need to experience reality in ways determined by his past will have been transformed into a capacity to know and to accept reality as it is, the hallmark of mental health.

WHAT IS THE RELATIONSHIP BETWEEN EMPATHY AND PROJECTIVE IDENTIFICATION?

It was only recently that I came to understand an important relationship between the deficiency-compensation model and the relational-conflict model. It has to do with the empathic failures of self psychology (a deficiency-compensation model).

I knew that, inevitably, narcissistic (or positive) transferences were disrupted by the therapist's empathic failures. I knew that the therapist was thought to have failed a patient empathically when the therapist failed to perform the selfobject function assigned him by the patient. But I had assumed that such failures were more or less random events—that a punctual therapist who had never been late might one day be late, which would be devastating for the patient, or that a therapist who was not ordinarily critical might one day say something that either seemed to the patient to be critical or was actually critical, which would also be devastating for the patient.

Now, however, I am coming to understand that, in fact, the therapist's so-called inevitable empathic failures are not random events but are very much determined by the patient's history. In other words, the therapist's failures are specific events that relate directly to the patient's history.

The therapist will fail the patient repeatedly, will make many mistakes. But the mistakes that the patient picks up on (and experiences as devastatingly unempathic) will be ones that the patient is particularly sensitized to because of his early-on history.

Furthermore, because of the interpersonal pressure exerted by the patient on the therapist to become the bad parent the patient had, the therapist may unwittingly accept the patient's projections — which will put the therapist in the position of failing the patient in ways specifically determined by the patient's history. In other words, the patient's need to have the therapist be the bad parent he had puts the therapist at risk for failing the patient in exactly those ways that the patient needs to be failed. In fact, we could think of the therapist's failures as arising from the therapist's empathic attunement to what the patient most needs.

The patient's need to re-create his past in the present (a compulsive repetition) has both an unhealthy component and a healthy component. The unhealthy piece has to do with the patient's need to re-create more of same because that is all the patient has ever known, and the healthy piece has to do with the patient's need to re-create more of same in the hope that this time the outcome will be different, the resolution a healthier one; first more of same and then something better; first bad and then bad made good. And so the therapist's failing the patient in ways specifically determined by the patient's history offers the patient an opportunity to achieve belated mastery.

I am speaking, then, to the connection between the deficiency-compensation model of self psychology, which places in the limelight the therapist's inevitable empathic failures (or optimal disillusionments), and the relational-conflict model, which involves the patient's re-creation in the here and now of the early-on traumatic failure situation in the hope that the resolution this time will be different. This is the relationship between empathic failure and projection/projective identification, the relationship between positive transference disrupted and negative transference.

Winnicott (1963b) captures beautifully the essence of this when he writes:

> Corrective provision is never enough. . . . In the end the patient uses the analyst's failures, often quite small ones, perhaps manoeuvred by the patient. . . . The operative factor is that the patient now hates the analyst for the failure that originally came as an environmental factor, outside the infant's area of omnipo-

tent control but that is now staged in the transference. So in the end we succeed by failing — failing the patient's way. This is a long distance from the simple theory of cure by corrective experience. [p. 258]

In the end, the therapist fails the patient in the ways that the patient's parent had failed him. It is important that we allow the patient to make us fail him in such ways. The patient choreographs our moves, and we dance them.

The patient's upset has to do with both his experience of the therapist as indeed the bad parent he had (negative transference) and his experience of the therapist as not the good parent he would have wished to have (positive transference disrupted). It is therefore doubly painful for the patient.

But, as part of the grieving process, the patient both comes to terms with the reality of the therapist's (and, before him, the parent's) very real limitations and comes to understand his own investment in getting his objects to fail him, his compulsive need to re-create with his contemporary objects the early-on traumatic failure situation.

As part of working through the therapist's failures of the patient, the patient has an opportunity both to add new good structure and to modify existent pathological structure.

WHY IS IT SO DIFFICULT FOR THE THERAPIST TO GET IT JUST RIGHT?

If therapists never allow themselves to be drawn into participating with patients in their reenactments, then we speak of a failure of empathy. On the other hand, if therapists allow themselves to be drawn into their patients' internal dramas but then get lost in the reenactment, then we speak of a failure of containment.

It is such a fine line that the therapist must tread. On the one hand, the therapist must have the capacity to respond empathically to the patient's need to be failed, the patient's transferential need to have the therapist be the old bad object. On the other hand, the therapist must also have the capacity to provide containment, to step back from his participation in the reenactment so that the response the therapist provides will be, ultimately, a corrective one.

TWELVE

The Attainment of Mature Hope

HOW IS UNREALISTIC HOPE TRANSFORMED INTO REALISTIC HOPE?

The process of structural growth and change is accompanied by the transformation of unrealistic hope into realistic hope, infantile hope into mature hope. Infantile hope relates to the patient's wish for his objects to be other than who they are; infantile hope, therefore, is pathological. According to Harold Searles (1979), mature hope arises in the context of surviving the experience of disappointment; mature hope, therefore, is a hallmark of mental health.

Mature hope emerges as a consequence of confronting certain intolerably painful realities head on and discovering that one survives the experience. It is by way of facing his disappointment—and finding that he survives it—that the patient is able to find his way to a healthy capacity for hope, based on realistic aspirations. The mature hope that results from the experience of mastering disenchantment has to do with attaining something that is realizable. By having the experience of grief and discovering that he can triumph over it, the patient wends his way toward health.

As Searles (1979) has written, "A healthy capacity for hope is founded . . . in past experiences of the successful integrating of disappointments—past experiences, that is, of successful grieving" (p. 483).

As the patient finally confronts the reality of the parental limitations, he lets go of the defenses around which the resistance has organized itself. As he discovers that he survives his confrontations with reality, the defenses to which he has clung since earliest childhood in order to protect him from knowing become ever less necessary.

As the resistance is overcome, the patient becomes freer to feel/do what he knows he should feel/do. He lets go of a past that has restricted his choices and embraces a present that offers an abundance of possibilities. Transformation of energy into structure, need into capacity, as the need to experience reality in ways determined by the past, becomes transformed into a capacity to know and to accept reality as it is.

Within the context of the safety provided by the relationship with his therapist, the patient is able at last to feel the pain he has spent a lifetime defending himself against. Transformation of infantile hope into mature hope results from the surviving of that pain; by having the experience of grief and discovering that he can triumph over it, the patient finds his way toward realistic hope and health.

References

Angyal, A. (1965). *Neurosis and Treatment: A Holistic Theory.* New York, London: John Wiley.
Baker, H. S., and Baker, M. N. (1987). Heinz Kohut's self psychology: an overview. *American Journal of Psychiatry* 144:1-9.
Balint, M. (1968). *The Basic Fault: Therapeutic Aspects of Regression.* New York: Brunner/Mazel.
Bibring, E. (1953). The mechanism of depression. In *Affective Disorders,* ed. P. Greenacre, pp. 154-181. New York: International Universities Press.
Buber, M. (1966). *Tales of the Hasidim: The Early Masters.* New York: Schocken Books.
Fairbairn, W. R. D. (1943). The repression and the return of bad objects. In *An Object-Relations Theory of the Personality,* pp. 59-81. New York: Basic Books, 1954.
_____ (1954). *An Object-Relations Theory of the Personality.* New York: Basic Books.
Freud, S. (1917). Mourning and melancholia. *Standard Edition* 14:237-260.
_____ (1923). The ego and the id. *Standard Edition* 19:1-66.
_____ (1926). Inhibitions, symptoms and anxiety. *Standard Edition* 20:77-175.
Gill, M. (1982). *Analysis of Transference,* vol. 1. New York: International Universities Press.

——— (1983). The interpersonal paradigm and the degree of the therapist's involvement. *Contemporary Psychoanalysis* 19:200–237.

Greenberg, J. R. (1986). Theoretical models and the analyst's neutrality. *Contemporary Psychoanalysis* 22:87–106.

Greenson, R. R. (1967). *The Technique and Practice of Psychoanalysis,* vol. 1. London: Hogarth.

Guntrip, H. (1973). *Psychoanalytic Theory, Therapy, and the Self.* New York: Basic Books.

Hartmann, H. (1939). *Ego Psychology and the Problem of Adaptation.* New York: International Universities Press.

Kernberg, O. F. (1976). *Object Relations and Clinical Psychoanalysis.* New York: Jason Aronson.

Klein, M. (1964). *Contributions to Psychoanalysis—1921–1945.* New York: McGraw-Hill.

——— (1975). *Envy and Gratitude and Other Works—1946–1963.* New York: Delacorte.

Kohut, H. (1966). Forms and transformations of narcissism. *Journal of the American Psychoanalytic Association* 14:243–257.

——— (1971). *The Analysis of the Self.* New York: International Universities Press.

——— (1977). *The Restoration of the Self.* New York: International Universities Press.

Kohut, H., and Wolf, E. (1978). The disorders of the self and their treatment: an outline. *International Journal of Psycho-Analysis* 59:413–425.

Kopp, S. (1969). The refusal to mourn. *Voices* Spring:30–35.

Kris, A. O. (1977). Either-or dilemmas. *Psychoanalytic Study of the Child* 32:91–117. New Haven, CT: Yale University Press.

Levenson, E. (1983). *The Ambiguity of Change.* New York: Basic Books.

Loewald, H. (1960). On the therapeutic action of psychoanalysis. *International Journal of Psycho-Analysis* 58:463–472.

Meissner, W. W. (1976). Psychotherapeutic schema based on the paranoid process. *International Journal of Psychoanalytic Psychotherapy* 5:87–113.

——— (1980). The problem of internalization and structure formation. *International Journal of Psycho-Analysis* 61:237–248.

Menninger, K. (1958). *Theory of Psychoanalytic Technique.* New York: Basic Books.

Mitchell, S. (1988). *Relational Concepts in Psychoanalysis.* Cambridge, MA: Harvard University Press.

Modell, A. (1975). A narcissistic defense against affects and the illusion of self-sufficiency. *International Journal of Psycho-Analysis* 56:275–282.

Racker, H. (1968). *Transference and Countertransference.* New York: International Universities Press.

Russell, P. (1980). The theory of the crunch (unpublished manuscript).

——— (1982). Beyond the wish: further thoughts on containment (unpublished manuscript).

Sandler, J. (1987). *From Safety to Superego: Selected Papers of Joseph Sandler.* New York: Guilford.

Schafer, R. (1968). *Aspects of Internalization.* New York: International Universities Press.

REFERENCES

Searles, H. (1979). The development of mature hope in the patient-therapist relationship. In *Countertransference and Related Subjects: Selected Papers,* pp. 479-502. New York: International Universities Press.

Thompson, C. (1950). *Psychoanalysis: Evolution and Development.* New York: Grove Press.

Winnicott, D. W. (1958). *Collected Papers: Through Paediatrics to Psycho-Analysis.* London: Tavistock.

―――― (1960). The theory of the parent–infant relationship. In *The Maturational Processes and the Facilitating Environment,* pp. 37-55. New York: International Universities Press, 1965.

―――― (1963a). From dependence to independence in the development of the individual. In *The Maturational Processes and the Facilitating Environment,* pp. 83-99. New York: International Universities Press, 1965.

―――― (1963b). Dependence in infant-care, in child-care, and in the psycho-analytic setting. In *The Maturational Processes and the Facilitating Environment,* pp. 249-259. New York: International Universities Press, 1965.

―――― (1965). *The Maturational Processes and the Facilitating Environment.* New York: International Universities Press.

Index

Absence of good, presence of bad and distinction between, negative transference, 208–209
Abuse survivors
 bad object internalization and, 20, 66–67
 depression and, 67–68
Abusive relationship, therapist understanding of, conveyance to patient, 124–125
Affect, defense-against-affect conflict statement and, 119–121
Affective nonrelatedness
 defense of, 173–174
 working through of, 178
Aggression, bad object internalization, 56
Anality
 capacity and strivings of, 38–40

traumatic frustration of needs, 49–50
Angyal, A., 106
Anxiety
 conflict and, 6–7
 creation of, 12–13
 easing of, 13
 intrapsychic/intrapersonal anxiety
  creation of, 12–13
  distinction between, 13–14
 modification statement, utility of, 227–228
 optimal level of, 134–135
 therapeutic relationship and, 94
 titration of, 134
Attention
 directing of, 98–99
  inward and backward, 225
  outward, 226
 modification statement and, 161–163

Attention (*continued*)
  repetition compulsion and, 99
  therapist intervention and, 191
Autonomy, achievement of, 35

Bad object, fear of, reconciliation of patient's need for, 10
Bad object internalization. *See also* Traumatic frustration
  abuse survivors and, 20
  clinical relevance of, 56–57
  Fairbairn on, 57–58, 62–63
  Freud on, 61–62
  good object internalization (therapist role) and, 85
  nature of, 56
  pathogenic introjects, 59–60
  relationships between objects
    Fairbairn on, 65
    Freud on, 63–64
    Kernberg and Meissner on, 65–66
  resistance and, 59
  therapeutic intervention and, 83
Baker, M., 197
Balint, M., 85, 92–93
Benevolent containment, described, 181
Betrayal. *See* Seduction and betrayal situation
Bibring, E., 44
Borderline patient
  conflict and, 140
  containing statement and, 140–141
Buber, M., 25–26

Capacity
  anal strivings and, 38–40
  for conflict statement
    described, 138–139
    example of lacking capacity, 138–139
  described, 37
  development of, 45–46
  Fairbairn on, 53–54
  for internalization, separateness and, 194–196
  object relations theory and, 83–84
  oedipal strivings and, 40
  self psychology and, 34–35, 46, 83
  structural growth and structural change, relationship between, 209
  traumatic frustration and, 52–53
Change
  agent of, therapeutic relationship, 211–212
  insight and, 225–226
Child abuse survivors. *See* Abuse survivors
Cocoon transference, 171–178
Compensation statement, described, 148–149
Conflict
  borderline patient and, 140
  clinical manifestation of, 3–4
  convergent conflict, experience of, 8
  convergent versus divergent, 7–8, 69
  descriptions of, 12
  ego defense and, 5
  examples of, 4, 5–6
  forces involved in, 6–7
  initial treatment stages, 174
  locus of, conflict statement and, 112–114
  operationalization of concept, 5
  patient awareness of, therapist intervention and, 118
  psychoanalytic conceptualization of (classic), 4
  reality and defense, 14
  situations of, 101–102
  therapist stance, 123–124
  traumatic frustration and, 69–70
  two-person psychology concept of, 68–69
Conflict statement. *See also entries under specific types of statements*
  compensation statement, 148–149
  confrontational, examples of, 132–133
  damaged-for-life statement, 147–148
  defense-against-affect conflict statement
    affect and, 119–121

INDEX

examples of, 115–117
experience and knowledge, 121
function of, 114–115
function of (first part), 117
function of (second part), 117–118
empowerment and, 122
entitlement statement, 149–150
examples of, resistance supporting,
   105–106
facilitation statement compared and
   contrasted, 167–168
function of, 104–105, 130, 132,
   142–143
illusion statement
   described, 152–153
   function of, 153–154
inverted conflict statement,
   described, 135–136
locus of conflict and, 112–114
modification statement and, 163–164
paradox, examples of, 133–134
path-of-least-resistance statement,
   described, 143–145
patient capacity for
   described, 138–139
   example of lacking capacity,
      139–140
patient response to
   defenses, 130–132
   optimal, 125–126
structure of, 122–123
types of, 126–127
work-to-be-done conflict statement
   described, 127
   function of, 129–130, 177–178
Confrontation
   conflict statement and, 132
   conflict statement examples and,
      132–133
Containing statement
   described, 140–141
   function of, 141–142
Containment failure, empathic failure
   and, therapeutic relationship, 234
Containment wishes, repetition
   compulsion and, 23
Convergent conflict

divergent conflict versus, 7–8, 69
experience of, 8
Corrective experience, insight and,
   therapist intervention, 212–213
Countertransference, projective
   identification and, relationship to
   projection and transference,
   218–219

Damaged-for-life statement, described,
   147–148
Decentering, therapeutic relationship,
   96
Defense-against-affect conflict
   statement
   affect and, 119–121
   examples of, 115–117
   experience and knowledge, 121
   function of, 114–115
      first part, 117
      second part, 117–118
Defense-against-reality conflict
   statement, described, 126
Defense of relentless entitlement,
   described, 189
Defenses
   of affective nonrelatedness, 173–174
   challenge of, 102
   conflict and, 14
   ego-dystonic dynamic of, 231
   naming of, patient stance and,
      106–107
   needs for, failure to grieve and, 21
   object need, patient's denial of,
      therapist response to, 174–175
   patient investment in, therapist
      acknowledgment of, 175
   reality and, 126
   relinquishment of
      patient requirements for, 128–129
      transference, 31
   resistance and, 14–15
   support of, 102–103
      challenge combined with, 103–104,
         136–137
      example of, 108, 110–112

Deficiency-compensation model, described, 85-86
Deficit development, traumatic frustration and, 52-53
Depression
  bad object internalization and, 67-68
  empty depression, described, 44
Direct transference, described, 74
Disappointment, reality of parental limitations, 19-20
Disillusionment. *See also* Parental failures and limitations
  benevolent containment and, 181
  grieving process and, 205-206
  integration statement, utility of, 203
  internal self regulation, transference and, 41-42
  nontraumatic (optimal) versus traumatic, 35-36
  seduction and betrayal situation and, 201-202
  working through of, 190-191
Disillusion statement
  described, 154-155
  as legitimization statement, 155
  utility of, 202-203
Disrupted positive transference, described, 196-197
Distortion
  described, 8-9
  patient investment in, 9-10
  therapeutic relationship and, 150-152
  toxic failures create need for, 20-21
  transference and, 9
Distortion statement
  described, 157-159
  utility of, 223-224
Divergent conflict, convergent conflict versus, 7-8, 69
Drives
  id, mastery of, results, 40
  internal drive regulation
    description of, 38
    self psychology and, 38
Drive theory
  conflict and, 4
  convergent versus divergent conflict, 7-8
  infantile need, 48

Ego
  defenses
    conflict and, 5
    ego-dystonic dynamic of, 231
  need (of patient), id versus ego needs, 182
  synthetic function of, 231
  therapeutic relationship and, 94-95, 98
Empathic failure
  containment failure and, therapeutic relationship, 234
  integration statement, described, 155-157
  location of, 198
  misperception and, 199-200
  therapist responsibility in, 198-199
Empathy
  easy versus difficult, 96-97
  listening, therapeutic relationship, 91-99
  meaning of, 97-98
  projective identification and, 232-234
Empowerment
  conflict statement and, 122
  structural growth and, 211
  techniques of, 107-108
  of therapist by patient, 172-173
Empty depression, described, 44. *See also* Depression
Entitlement
  defense of relentless entitlement, described, 189
  narcissistic transference and, 187-188
  therapeutic relationship and, 150-152
Entitlement statement
  described, 149-150
  function of, 188
  working through and, 190-191

INDEX

Experience
  defense-against-affect conflict statement, 121
  negative filters and, 222-223
Experience-near therapist intervention, described, 121
Experiencing ego, therapeutic relationship and, 94-95

Facilitation statement
  conflict statement and, 167-168
  described, 165-167
  function of, 176
Failure (by therapist), trauma and, 186. *See also* Empathic failure
Failure to grieve
  defense needs and, 21
  internal impoverishment and, 26
  patient's refrain when experiencing, 26-27
  resistance and, 19-28
Fairbairn, W. R. D., 53-54, 55, 57-58, 59, 60, 62-63, 65, 66
Fear, negative transference and, 79
Freud, S., 4, 60, 61-62, 63-64, 65, 66

Gill, M., 85
Good object internalization (therapist role)
  bad object internalization and, 85
  dynamics of, 230
  need for, and old bad object, 87
Greenberg, J., 87
Greenson, R., 4, 220
Grieving process
  described, 24-25
  disillusionment and, 205-206
  empathy and projective identification, 234
  failure to grieve. *See* Failure to grieve
  internalization and, 30-31
  negative transference resolution and, 230-231
  parental failures and limitations and, 30
  patient needs in, 203-204
  pseudo-grief, described, 25-26
  repetition compulsion and, 24
  resistance mastered by, 29-32
  treatment situation creates opportunity for, 24
  working through, transference, 31-32
Guilt, bad object internalization and, 67-68
Guntrip, H., 85

Hartmann, H., 35
Health. *See* Mental health
Hope
  attainment of, 235-236
  positive transference and, 78-79

Id
  mastery of, results, 40
  need (of patient), id versus ego needs, 182
Idealizing transference, described, 81-82
Illusion
  described, 8-9
  narcissistic transference and, 185
  needs for, perfection needs and, 45
  patient investment in, 9-10
  therapeutic relationship and, 150-152
  toxic failures create need for, 20-21
  transference and, 9
Illusion statement
  described, 152-153
  function of, 153-154, 186-187
  working through and, 190-191
Impasse. *See* Therapeutic impasse
Infantile need
  described, 48
  examples of, 48
Insight
  change and, 225-226
  corrective experience and, therapist intervention, 212-213
  as corrective for transference distortion, 213-214

Integration statement
  described, 155–157
  utility of, 203
Internal drive regulation
  description of, 38
  self psychology and, 38
Internal impoverishment, failure to grieve and, 26
Internalization
  of bad object, 20. *See also* Bad object internalization
  capacity for, separateness and, 194–196
  Fairbairn on, 53–54
  grieving process and, 30–31
  process of, 35
  reality versus perfectionism, 43–44
  separation process and, 55–56
  traumatic frustration and, 51–52, 53
Internal self regulation
  self psychology and, 41
  transference and, 41–42
Interpersonal anxiety, creation of, 12–13. *See also* Anxiety
Interpersonal relations, abuse. *See* Abusive relationship
Interpretation
  positive transference and, 193–194
  of transference, 79–80
Intervention. *See* Therapeutic relationship; Therapist intervention
Intrapsychic anxiety, creation of, 12–13. *See also* Anxiety
Inverted conflict statement, described, 135–136
Inverted modification statement, utility of, 228–229
Inverted transference
  described, 74
  example of, 75
  projection and projective identification related to, 220–221

Kernberg, O., 60, 65–66
Klein, M., 84, 216

Knowledge
  conflict statement and, 122
  defense-against-affect conflict statement, 121
Kohut, H., 41, 54, 55, 67, 85, 194–195
Kopp, S., 27, 30, 204, 205
Kris, A. O., 7

Legitimization statement
  described, 159–160
  disillusion statement, described, 154–155
  function of, 176–177, 189–190
  utility of, 224–225
  working through and, 190–191
Levenson, E., 85
Libido, bad object internalization, 56
Listening, therapeutic relationship, 91–99
Locus
  conflict statement, locus of conflict and, 112–114
  negative transference, 222
Loewald, H., 85

Mastery, nontraumatic (optimal) disillusionment and, 55
Mature capacity. *See* Capacity
Mature hope, attainment of, 235–236
Meissner, W. W., 60, 65–66, 85
Menninger, K., 96, 99
Mental health
  described, 11–12
  self psychology and, 36–37, 206
  transference resolution and, 32
Mental illness, pathogenesis, 47–71. *See also* Bad object internalization
Mitchell, S., 68–69, 85
Modell, A., 173
Modification statement
  conflict statement and, 163–164
  described, 161–163
  inverted, 164–165
  utility of, 227–228

Narcissistic demands, therapist compliance with, 192–193

INDEX

Narcissistic development, 42–43
Narcissistic needs
  described, 51
  traumatic frustration of, 50–51
Narcissistic patient, with structural deficit, presentation of, 183–184
Narcissistic rage, described, 197
Narcissistic transference
  entitlement and, 187–188
  illusion and, 185
  seduction and betrayal situation and, 201
Need (of patient)
  gratification of, necessary but not sufficient for growth, 193
  patient's denial of object need, therapist response to, 174–175
  perfection needs, positive transference and, 184
  psychological/physiological compared, 181–182
  respect for, and interpretation of, 109
Negative filters, self experience and, 222–223
Negative self perception, traumatic frustration and, 70–71
Negative transference, 207–234. *See also* Positive transference; Transference
  absence of good and presence of bad, distinction between, 208–209
  development of, 73–74
  direct transference, described, 74
  disrupted positive transference and, 80–81, 200
  distortion statement
    described, 157–159
    utility of, 223–224
  fear and, 79
  grieving process in resolution of, 230–231
  insight as corrective for transference distortion, 213–214
  interpretation and, 79–80
  inverted transference, described, 74
  legitimization statement, utility of, 224–225
  locus of, 222
  object relations theory and, 207–208, 216–218
  paradox and, 215–216
  positive transference and, 78
  recognition of, 218
  resolution of, 75
    one-person theory, 75–76
    two-person theory, 75–76
  structural growth and structural change, relationship between, 209
  therapeutic relationship and, 214–215, 221
Neurotic needs, described, 51
Nontoxic reality, toxic reality versus, 15–17
Nontraumatic (optimal) disillusionment
  mastery and, 55
  traumatic versus, 35–36
Nontraumatic (optimal) frustration
  mental health and, 47–48
  positive transference and, 180–181

Object relations theory
  bad object internalization, 56
  capacity and, 83–84
  negative transference and, 207–208, 216–218
Observing ego, therapeutic relationship and, 94–95, 98
Oedipal needs
  capacity and, 40
  traumatic frustration of, 50
One-person theory, negative transference resolution and, 75–76. *See also* Psychoanalysis (classic)
Optimal disillusionment. *See* Nontraumatic (optimal) disillusionment

Paradox
  conflict statement and, 132
  conflict statement examples, 133–134

Paradox (*continued*)
  negative transference and, 215–216
  positive transference and, 204–205
  working through, transference, defense relinquishment and, 31
Parental failures and limitations. *See also* Disillusionment
  grieving process and, 30
  reality and, 19–20
Path-of-least-resistance statement, described, 143–145
Pathogenesis, 47–71. *See also* Bad object internalization; Traumatic frustration
Pathogenic introjects, described, 59–60
Perception, reality and, 8
Perfectionism, reality versus, internalization, 43–44
Perfection needs
  developmental processes and, 42
  illusion needs and, 45
  positive transference and, 184
Perfect object need, developmental processes and, 42–43
Positive transference, 179–206. *See also* Negative transference; Transference
  disrupted, 196–197
    locating of, 198
    misperception and, 199–200
    negative transference and, 80–81
    therapist responsibility in, 198–199
  emergence of, 179–180
  hope and, 78–79
  interpretation and, 79–80, 193–194
  negative transference and, 78
  paradox and, 204–205
  perfection needs and, 184
  seduction and betrayal situation and, 200–202
Power. *See* Empowerment
Presence of bad, absence of good and distinction between, negative transference, 208–209
Price-paid conflict statement
  described, 126
  function of, 127–128

Projection
  directing of, 219–220
  inverted transference and projective identification related to, 220–221
  transference and, relationship to projective identification and countertransference, 218–219
Projective identification
  countertransference and, relationship to projection and transference, 218–219
  directing of, 219–220
  empathy and, 232–234
  inverted transference and projection related to, 220–221
  transference and, 220
Pseudo-grief, described, 25–26
Psychic structure. *See* Capacity
Psychoanalysis (classic)
  agent of change in, 211
  bad object internalization and, 61–62
  conflict and, 4, 69
  drive theory and, 38
  one-person theory, 68

Racker, H., 85
Rage. *See* Narcissistic rage
Reality
  conflict and, 14
  conflict statements and, 126–127
  defenses and, 126
  grieving process and, 25
  of parental limitations, 19–20
  perception and, 8
  perfectionism versus, internalization, 43–44
  toxic versus nontoxic, 15–17
  transference and, 10–11
Relational-conflict model, described, 86–87
Repetition compulsion
  containment wishes and, 23
  described, 22
  doubled-edged nature of, 23–24
  grieving process and, 24
  patient's action and, 99

INDEX

patient's attention brought to, 99
power of, 22
traumatic frustration and, 77-78
Resistance
  bad object internalization and, 56, 59
  concept of, 3-17
  conflict statement supporting, examples of, 105-106
  defenses and, 14-15
  defined, 17
  failure to grieve and, 19-28
  mastery of, by grieving, 29-32
  patient rationale for, 173
  separation from infantile object in overcoming, 232
  transference and, 171-172
  working through of, described, 95
Russell, P., 22, 23, 24

Sandler, J., 85
Schafer, R., 60
Searles, H., 235-236
Second chance, meaning of, 185
Seduction and betrayal situation, positive transference and, 200-202
Self experience. *See* Experience
Self psychology
  capacity and, 46, 83
  described, 33-34
  grieving, internalization, and structuralization relationships in, 34-35
  internal drive regulation and, 38
  internal self regulation and, 41
  mental health and, 36-37, 206
  negative transference and, 207-208
  value of, 182-183
Separateness, capacity for internalization and, 194-196
Separation, from infantile object in overcoming resistance, 232
Separation process, internalization and, 55-56
Serial dilutions, described, 84

Sermonizing, therapeutic relationship and, 191-192
Structural change
  clinical examples of, 210-211
  structural growth and, relationship between, 209
Structural growth
  clinical examples of, 209
  empowerment and, 211
  structural change and, relationship between, 209
Structures. *See* Capacity
Suicide, listening and, 109

Therapeutic impasse
  example of, 146
  factors in, 27
  forces creating, 145
  interventions for, 146-147
Therapeutic relationship. *See also* Therapist intervention
  abusive relationship, therapist understanding of, conveyance to patient, 124-125
  agent of change in, 211-212
  anxiety
    optimal level of, 134-135
    titration of, 134
  conflict, therapist stance toward, 123-124
  deficiency-compensation model, 85-86
  empathic failure/containment failure, 234
  listening, 91-99
  narcissistic demands, therapist compliance with, 192-193
  negative transference and, 214-215, 221
  relational-conflict model, 86-87
  second chance, meaning of, 185
  sermonizing and, 191-192
  therapist as new good object, 230
Therapist intervention. *See also* Therapeutic relationship
  attention and, 191
  bad object internalization and, 83

Therapist intervention (*continued*)
  conflict, patient awareness of, 118
  defenses, object need, patient's denial of, therapist response to, 174–175
  experience-near, 121
  individual style in, 137–138
  insight and corrective experience, 212–213
  therapeutic impasse, 146–147
Thompson, C., 230
Toxic reality, nontoxic reality versus, 15–17
Transference. *See also* Narcissistic transference; Negative transference; Positive transference
  cocoon transference, 171–178
  directing of, 219–220
  idealizing transference, described, 81–82
  illusion and distortion in, 9
  interpretation of, 79–80
  narcissistic transference, illusion and, 185
  projection and, relationship to projective identification and countertransference, 218–219
  projective identification and, 220
  reality and, 10–11
  resistance and, 171–172
  resolution of, mental health and, 32
  traumatic frustration and, 77–78
  working through
    defense relinquishment and, 31
    grieving process and, 31–32
    internal self regulation and, 41–42
    results of, 44–45
  working with, 73–87
Trauma, failure (by therapist) and, 186
Traumatic disillusionment, nontraumatic (optimal) versus, 35–36

Traumatic frustration. *See also* Bad object internalization
  of anal needs, 49–50
  conflict and, 69–70
  deficit development and, 52–53
  internalization and, 51–52
  internal records of, 77
  mental illness and, 47–48
  of narcissistic needs, 50–51
  negative self perception and, 70–71
  of oedipal needs, 50
  positive transference and, 180–181
  results of, 49
  summary of sequelae of, 54
  transference and, 77–78
Two-person psychology
  agent of change and, 212
  conflict and, 68–69
  negative transference resolution and, 75–76

Unrealistic hope, attainment of, 235–236

Winnicott, D. W., 92–93, 182, 194–195, 217, 233–234
Wolf, E., 85
Working through
  of affective nonrelatedness, 178
  of disillusionment, 190–191
  disillusionment statement, utility of, 202–203
  object relations theory and, 216–218
  of resistance, described, 95
  transference
    defense relinquishment and, 31
    grieving process and, 31–32
    self psychology and, 83
Work-to-be-done conflict statement
  described, 127
  function of, 129–130, 177–178